Stem Cells, Exosomes and Beyond

The who, what, how, and why of Regenerative Biologics

THIRD EDITION

by

Dmitry M Arbuck, MD

To my family and friends whose time I borrowed to write this book

Stem Cells, Exosomes and Beyond

The who, what, how, and why of Regenerative Biologics

THIRD EDITION

by

Dmitry M Arbuck, MD

Copyright © 2022 by AMEI

All rights reserved. No part of this book shall be reproduced, stored in a retrieval system, or transmitted by any means, electronic, mechanical, photocopying, recording or otherwise, without written permission from the publisher. No liability is assumed with respect to the use of the information contained herein. Although every precaution has been taken in the preparation of this book, the publisher and author assume no responsibility for errors and omissions. Nor is any liability assumed for damages resulting from the use of the information contained herein.

ISBN 978-1-7341237-3-9

1. Medicine. 2. Health.

Printed in the United States of America

Third Edition, Printed June 2022

Second Edition, Printed October 2020

First Printing October 2019

Warning and Disclaimer

This book is not intended as a substitute for the medical advice of a physician. The reader should regularly consult a physician in matters relating to his or her health and particularly with respect to any symptoms that may require diagnosis or medical attention.

Image Credits

Many images in this book have been donated, these are credited below the image. Other images have been used under license from Shutterstock.com and Vectorstock.com.

Bulk Sales

Please contact us at amei@solucid.com and we will be happy to discuss your bulk purchase needs.

Managing Editor

Paul Adams

"Surely every medicine is an innovation,

and he that will not apply new remedies must expect new evils"

Sir Francis Bacon, 1561-1626

"You will observe with concern how long a useful truth may be known and exist

before it is generally received and practiced on"

Benjamin Franklin, 1706-1790

TABLE OF CONTENTS

1   Introduction
4   Stem cell deification
5   Who is this book for?

PART ONE: WHAT ARE STEM CELLS?

8   What are stem cells?
8   A brief history of stem cells
9   What do stem cells do?
10   What happens to stem cells in the body?
11   Stem cell life cycle
13   Cell hierarchy
14   How are stem cells collected?
15   Autologous and allogeneic stem cells
16   Mesenchymal and hematopoietic stem cells
19   Fetal wound healing
20   Amniotic and umbilical stem cell products
22   Cellular and extracellular products
24   Telomeres and aging
26   Estimating the number of cells
27   Exosomes
31   Animal stem cell products

PART TWO: PROBLEMS & CONCERNS

34   Stem cell problems and concerns
34   Risks of stem cell treatment
34   Religious concerns
35   Embryonic stem cells
36   Umbilical cord stem cells
36   Induced pluripotent stem cells
37   Overseas stem cell treatment
38   Regulation
41   What is prohibited?
42   Donating stem cells & to whom they belong
44   Donor and tissue screening
44   Testing and counting cells
45   Vitality and preservation
47   Graft-versus-host disease
47   Opening the blood-brain barrier
48   Host DNA replacement by donor DNA

PART THREE: CLINICAL APPLICATIONS

52   The clinical applications of stem cells
52   Patient experience

54	Post-treatment guidelines
55	Duration of stem cell action
55	What about multiple conditions?
56	Stem cells and medications
56	Intravenous administration
58	Epidural injections
59	Intrathecal stem cells
59	Intraarticular administration
61	Intradiscal injections
63	Intramuscular injections
64	Intraligament injections
64	Intraosseous injections
65	Intracardiac injections
65	Intraorgan injections
65	Brain and intraspinal treatments
68	Intraocular and eye surface treatment
68	Intranasal treatment
69	Stem cells and cancer
69	Can stem cells be used to treat pain?
70	Dental applications
71	Cosmetic treatment
72	Hair color
72	Can stem cells prolong life?
73	Growing organs
73	Scar formation
74	Mental illness
74	Stem cells and COVID
77	Other regenerative medicine products
77	Emerging stem cell related products
78	Examples of acellular products
80	Cord blood vs. tissue allografts
81	Conclusion

PART FOUR: END MATTER

84	Appendix 1: Selected Stem Cell Glossary
85	Appendix 2: Notable Dates
86	Appendix 3: Amniotic Product Components
87	Appendix 4A: Growth Regulating Factors
88	Appendix 4B: Immune Regulating Factors
89	Appendix 5: Section 351 vs. 361 Flowchart
90	Appendix 6: Stem Cell Based Product Classifications
91	Appendix 7: Post Treatment Instructions
92	Appendix 8: Placental-Derived Tissue Components
93	Appendix 9: Current Stem Cell Studies
93	Acknowledgments
94	Endnotes
106	Index

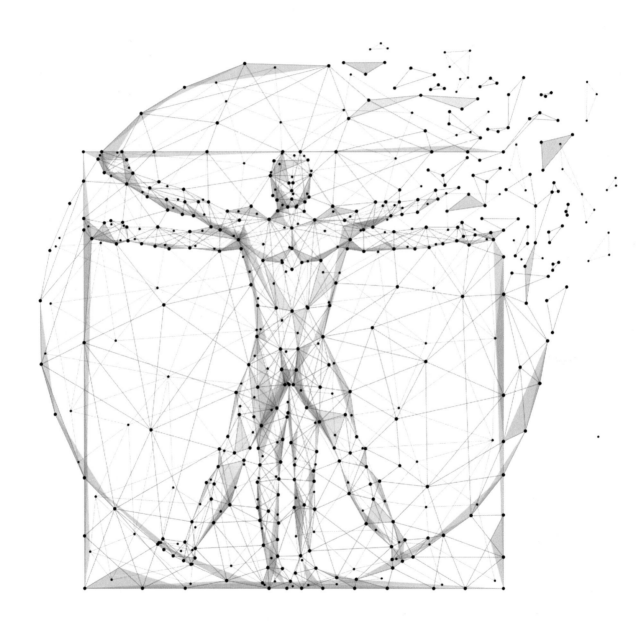

Introduction

Our personal experiences define what we trust and apply to our lives; this is especially true with controversial subjects where a commonly accepted opinion does not exist.

Stem cells and regenerative medicine have intrigued me for a long time. Most pharmaceutical treatments seek to maintain the status quo. We have sophisticated tools to keep blood pressure down, suppress the immune system, control arthritis inflammation, etc. These medications may afford the patient a comfortable life but fail to deliver a cure. With few exceptions, the health care system attends to the symptoms of diseases and disorders without eliminating their cause. Regenerative medicine, especially stem cell based treatments offer a new opportunity to enhance an efficient self-repair system far beyond an aging body's natural capacity. What a welcome development!

In the early 2000s, I flew to Germany to learn about stem cells. The technology was in its infancy at that time. Researchers took questionable paths, working with animal and human embryonic stem cells, a practice that evoked strong and understandable objections. Stem cells harvested from patients were collected through invasive and sometimes painful procedures. Manipulation of cells outside of the body, conducted without established and safe technologies, also caused problems. Many of the products labeled "stem cells" were not stem cells. If they were, the cells were often dead on arrival.

Clearly, stem cells were not ready for clinical practice in the United States. I returned home, determined to keep an eye on ongoing developments. In 2016, I became aware that several US labs had started to offer umbilical cord stem cells. These young, neutral, reportedly safe cells seemed to hold real clinical promise.

The timing was right for me. For two years, I had suffered from a severe autoimmune skin condition. I had an intolerable rash that burned, itched, and constantly left me with painful broken skin. It made my life miserable. I lost 30 pounds and could not sleep. My legs would swell, making walking painful, and made my gums bleed due to autoimmune damage. I went through the day weak and dizzy. A whole gamut of other non-specific symptoms plagued me. No treatment helped. The only remedy that provided some relief was injections of high dose steroids. The rash often covered so much of my body that the nurse had difficulty finding a place to stick a needle. Without another choice for treatment,

I exceeded the annual steroid dose by three times. What else could I do? Oral steroids did not work. Injections provided two weeks of relative improvement at most before the symptoms returned with a vengeance. Cancer and rheumatologic immunosuppressive treatments were not palatable to me.

Stem cell treatment, which would disrupt my condition at its root cause, seemed the only reasonable solution. I looked into the suppliers and some bad actors set alarm bells ringing. After a thorough vetting process, I identified a lab that offered high-quality umbilical blood stem cells. I made a trip to see the facility and meet the team. I discussed the latest developments with the scientists and saw the actual process of stem cell examination.

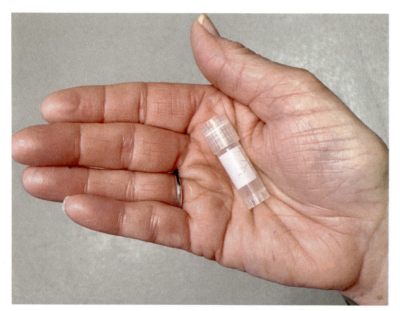

A stem cell vial on my assistant's palm

Everything seemed to be falling in place. I had a ready patient: myself and I had enough knowledge to recognize that the benefits of using stem cells likely outweighed the risks.

Understandably, I was anxious. As a physician, I do not want to cause harm to any patient, including myself. Stem cells made sense theoretically, but even the soundest medical theories require practical grounding. Book learning cannot replace solid clinical judgment. I had to either take a risk by treating my intractable condition with stem cells or continue hurting myself with the steroids and oher immunosuppressants – known treatments, though, in my case, ineffective and dangerous in the long run.

The day came and I thawed a frozen cell vial in the palm of my hand. The contents were infused into my vein. And nothing happened. I felt absolutely nothing. I did not know what that night would bring. Would I have a stroke? Would I turn into some deformed creature? Would I grow a third eye? Fortunately, none of the above. The next day was my day off. That evening, I received a call from Paul, the CEO of my clinic. He asked how I felt and I shrugged and replied, "I feel nothing." We kept discussing the treatment, and it suddenly occurred to me that I actually felt nothing. No burning, no itching. None. Zilch. And my rash was pale.

By the end of the next day, 90% of my rash had disappeared. You can imagine how I felt. It felt really good. Unbelievable, maybe! I had a second treatment two weeks later. After a few days, my rash was about 98% gone. I had an exacerbation in three months. Another treatment took care of my symptoms for six months. Each time my symptoms returned, they were less severe. My fourth and last treatment seemed to take care of my mysterious autoimmune disease, and I am now almost symptom-free for several years. I regained weight and no longer needed to avoid foods, detergents, wool, or the other things I had cut out of my life. If my symptoms decide to come back, I know what to do. I am not cured; I still have a rash at times, but only mild and local, a far cry from the original disease.

In my practice, I treat patients with chronic painful conditions. Many of them have illnesses that do not respond to conventional treatment. My successful self-treatment gave me the courage to offer similar treatments to my patients. I am still surprised by how many remarkable results and otherwise impossible outcomes these unproven therapies deliver. Stem cell treatments have restored my long-suffering patients' knees, shoulders, necks, and low backs. I have been thanked for curing lungs, kidneys, the gut, and autoimmune diseases. I have seen wounds and resistant infections heal, brain function improve, and hearts rid themselves of post-myocardial infarction scars. Many patients, rescued from chronic pain, got off their daily medications and returned to a fulfilling life.

Umbilical cord wall and umbilical cord blood stem cells are still a novelty and there is much more work to be done before they are widely adopted for clinical use. Hidden dangers may later surface. But at least an alternative was available for patients who have exhausted conventional treatments for otherwise incurable conditions. As regenerative medicine science develops, we learn more about stem cell components - exosomes, and specific active factors within exosomes. As our knowledge expands, more precision treatments become available.

Due to regulatory pressures, live stem cells are now very difficult, if not impossible, to obtain in the US. Cellular and acellular biological products derived from cord wall, amniotic fluid, and other live birth waste are currently available from a handful of labs. These other regenerative medicine products have most of the potential but are likely less powerful than live cells. We will talk about all of these regenerative products in this book.

I like to compare live stem cells to apple trees and exosomes (produced by stem cells) to the apples. Following this logic, growth factors and cytokines (contents of exosomes) are akin to fructose and vitamin C inside the apples. You may argue what is more important: the tree, the apple, or the juice, but all three are important in their own way.

After many years and thousands of treatments, many things became evident: Autoimmune conditions (including skin, gut, and multisystem) have the best response to treatment. Many joint treatments, including knee and shoulder, are easy and provide consistent and reliable results. Spinal disk treatments produce noticeable benefits in most patients. Less effective treatments include peripheral neuropathy and treatments for brain and spinal cord conditions. This unfortunate lack of efficacy may be caused by immature technology rather than an inability of regenerative medicine to treat such conditions. The simple truth is that panacea does not exist.

Throughout history, breakthrough health care technologies – immunizations, antiseptics, antibiotics, aspirin, MRI, and so on – have transformed medicine and bettered the lives of millions. We are standing on the doorstep of the next medical revolution with stem cells.

Stem cell deification

We love miracles. It is natural for people to want to see a miracle with regenerative treatments and this desire may blind people to trusting false claims that stem cells "cure" everything. Like everything else, they have their limitations.

If one's broken leg is surgically fixed, it does not mean that it cannot be broken again. Even if treatment helps, it does not mean that environmental or internal factors may not push a patient to another disease episode. It would be naive to expect a chronic severe, otherwise untreatable condition in an older individual to vanish without a trace after a single treatment. Not all conditions respond to treatments equally; the length of treatment and the doses vary depending on the individual circumstances. Thinking too well about stem cells is as bad as thinking of them *too* poorly.

Who is this book for?

When I set out to explore the potential of stem cell treatment about 20 years ago, there was no practical handbook for clinicians and their patients. As I wrote this book, it was still the case. *Stem Cell Solutions*, second edition, published in 2020, added specific treatment cases and scientific and COVID-related updates..

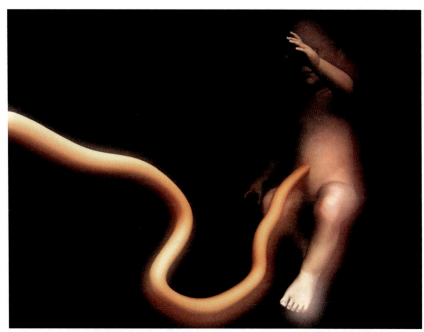
Umbilical cord stem cells come from the umbilical cord and other birth waste donated by healthy mothers after c-section childbirth.

This book addresses cellular and acellular stem cell related treatments, including extracellular matrix (fibers that aid in tissue regeneration) and more details about exosmes (vesicles produced stem cells and packaged with biologically active molecules). It also explains the recent significant regulatory changes in the United States. I hope this latest edition will help clinicians see the risks and rewards of bringing regenerative medicine into their practice. Likewise, I hope this book will improve the scientific literacy of patients seeking relief from intractable health problems and give them the tools they need to discern hucksters – of which there are many – from honest health care practitioners.

In the time since the second edition's publication, so much has changed that even the title had to be modified to underline the growing importance of acellular stem cell treatments. Stem Cells, Exosomes and Beyond covers the current state of the regenerative medicine.

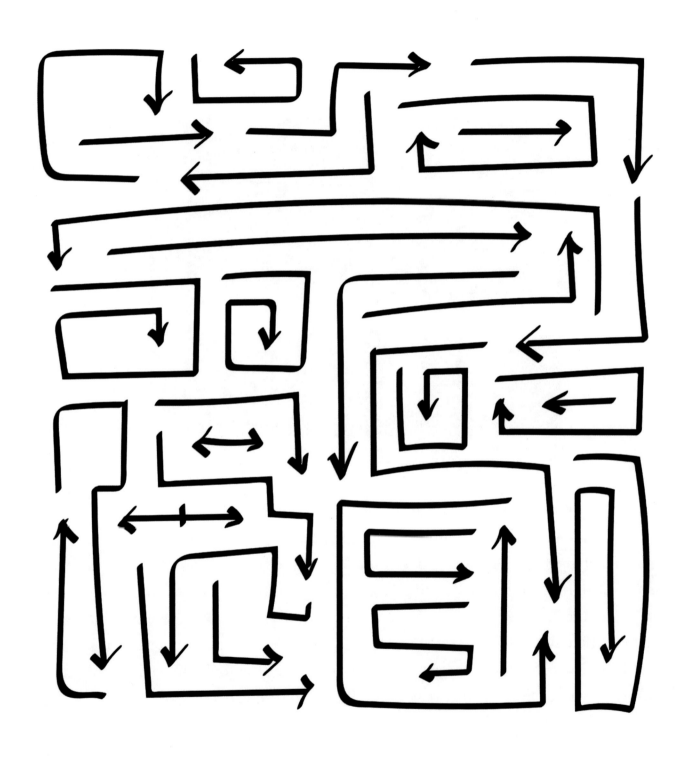

PART ONE:

WHAT ARE STEM CELLS?

What are stem cells?

Almost all tissues in the body contain stem cell populations. Stem cells may be considered the architects of every other cell. As such, they have the power to repair or rebuild damaged tissue. Successive generations of researchers and clinicians have undertaken the study of how to direct that power. Stem cells are powerhouses that produce many ingredients of life, and they have a reach well beyond the actual cell body. Below, we will review the most relevant issues surrounding stem cells.

A brief history of stem cells

The term "stammzelle" (German for stem cell) was first used by a German scientist Valentin Häcker in 1868. Following Häcker's work, in the early 1900's Russian micro-anatomist Alexander Maksimov and others used the term "stem cell" to explain hematopoiesis (how blood cells differentiate into their specialized roles). Through the second half of the twentieth century, researchers discovered stem cells in bone marrow, then umbilical cord blood. In 1981, the developmental biologist Gail Martin isolated stem cells from a mouse embryo at her lab at the University of California San Francisco. Since then, the sourcing and harvesting of stem cells have been widely diversified, often in response to religious or ethical concerns. Likewise, researchers have explored possible therapeutic applications for everything from autism to sickle cell anemia, from diabetes to autoimmune diseases. By 2017, over a million stem cell transplants had been recorded worldwide, and the number continues to grow. For more data points, see the timeline in "Appendix 2: Notable Dates" on page 85

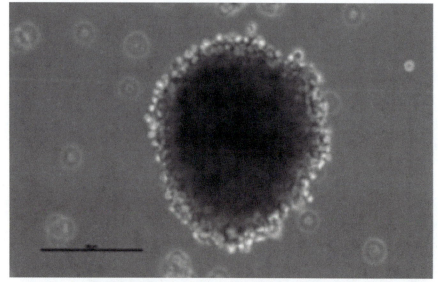

A stem cell 'sphere' that contains hundreds to thousands of stem cells, grown from a single cell – Courtesy Dr. W. Mark Erwin, University of Toronto

What do stem cells do?

In theory, transplanted stem cells should modify inflammation and repair damaged tissue. Although it is a necessary part of healing, unresolved inflammation in the body is catastrophic and, in one way or another, causes the majority of our diseases. Some conditions are broadly recognized as inflammatory: rheumatoid arthritis, asthma, Crohn's disease, inflammatory bowel disease, cancer, etc., are less intuitive, such as obesity or atherosclerosis.[1] In psychiatry, inflammation is associated with psychosis, autism, depression, and others.[2][3][4]

The potential for using regenerative products to disrupt the inflammatory process is vast. Immune regulating factors suppress inflammation and mobilize cells to the site of action. Although stem cell action is hypothesized to direct "healthy" inflammation where repair may occur in a more organized fashion, much remains to be determined.

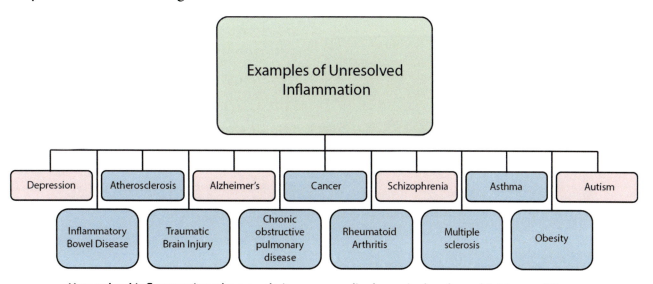

Unresolved inflammation plays a role in many medical, surgical and psychiatric conditions.

In addition, stem cells produce cytokines and growth factors, delivered by exosomes, involved in wound, heart, bone, nervous system, and other tissue healing (see "Exosomes" on page 27). Furthermore, stem cells may secrete free-floating active signaling molecules and fibrous elements, collectively called "matrix." Stem cells themselves can change their surroundings by immediate physical cell-to-cell interaction, and this cellular repair occurs through various mechanisms. Although the full spectrum of their curative properties remains unknown, there is evidence showing that stem cells heal, in part, through mitochondrial transfer, direct oxygen transmission from blood vessels to the tissues, and replacing damaged cells with healthy ones. These and other interactions, including specific secreted factors that travel from stem cells to other areas around the body, are explored throughout this text.

The regenerative potential of stem cells suggests surgical applications may be among the most common treatments, showing benefits before, during, and after surgery.[5][6] Applications of regenerative treatments in sports medicine are also widely known and publicized.

What happens to stem cells in the body?

Settling stem cells in the desired location within the body is called "homing." After intravenous infusion, the cells need to identify where to go and in which tissue to anchor. They seem to sense tissues and organs in distress. They probably have chemoreceptors that allow them to prioritize the risks to the patient's life. Stem cells will anchor (or "home") at the most urgent complaint. If a person suffers from heart disease and a muscle tear, intravenous stem cells would likely focus on the heart. In theory, when the heart is sufficiently repaired, they switch their attention to a peripheral problem.[7][8] When stem cells travel to the thymus, a major immune regulatory organ, they may help modulate the immune system.

> I have included several clinical case examples from my practice. These cases are not intended to suggest that patients with similar conditions would respond equally well to stem cell treatments. Please remember that no treatment, however advanced, guarantees improvement.

Transplanted stem cells have never been detected in a patient's body longer than a few weeks after the introduction. Much more research needs to be done to understand the survivability, destination, and influence of transplanted stem cells. If stem cells are injected peripherally (i.e., a joint), they mostly stay within the joint capsule and, therefore, local within the joint space. Soft tissue (muscle) injections allow more cells to be carried away to different body locations.

In addition to the cellular impact on the surrounding tissue, stem cells produce extracellular elements such as trophic factors, cytokines, and growth factors to influence the body after stem cell implantation. The clinical response to the treatment of autoimmune problems may be observed within 24 to 48 hours of treatment, while any potential tissue regeneration understandably requires more time.

Stem cell life cycle

Stem cells may replicate themselves or mature into specialized cells, effectively repairing injured organs. Through symmetric division, a stem cell divides into two identical stem cells.

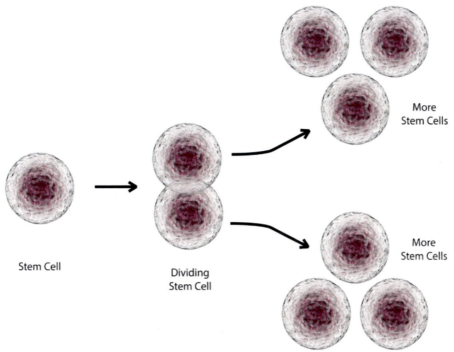

Symmetric division renders identical stem cells.

Through asymmetric division, a stem cell may divide into a copy of itself plus a specialized cell of adjacent tissue.[9,10,11,12,13]

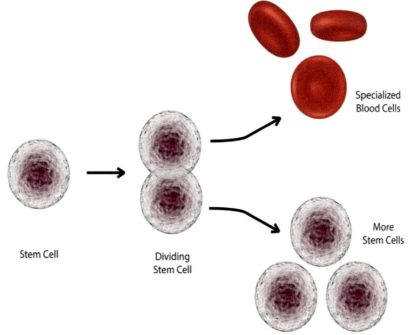

Asymmetric division yields stem cell replicas as well as specialized cells.

In addition to becoming mature tissue, stem cells can reprogram nearby sick or damaged cells by injecting them with healthy mitochondria and other inner cellular parts. This interaction between a stem cell and a cancer cell has been observed in a lab environment. Fatigued muscle, heart muscle, endocrine, and nerve tissue may be repaired similarly.[14] [15] [16] Whether stem cells consistently reprogram sick and damaged cells through such mitochondrial transfer remains unclear.[17]

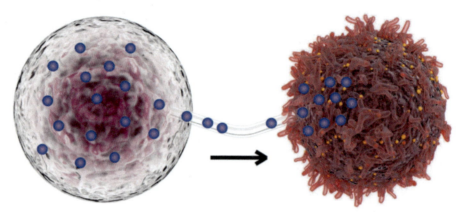

A stem cell delivers healthy mitochondria to a cancer cell.

Stem cells may position themselves on a blood vessel and transmit oxygen and nutrients to the suffering tissue. Even further, stem cells may ultimately form new blood vessels or repair damaged ones. Stem cells love oxygen, but they also increase tissue health by creating a better environment for themselves by improving vascularization.[18] [19] This is why introducing stem cells into poorly oxygenated areas of swelling or even into spinal discs may be beneficial. Even if stem cells die or disintegrate, their contents may still provide powerful healing properties.

Some types of stem cells can differentiate into nerve cells. One day, we may be able to place stem cells into a damaged brain or a nerve plexus to renew the area with young, new neurons.[20] [21] Such treatment remains in the realm of speculation for now.

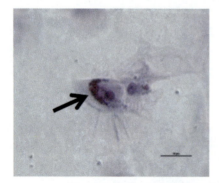 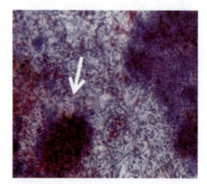 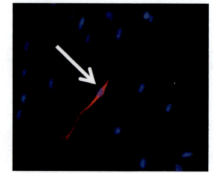

The same line of mesenchymal stem cells produced a fat cell (left), cartilage cell (middle), and bone cell (right). – Courtesy of Dr. W. Mark Erwin, University of Toronto

Cell hierarchy

Stem cells are popularly understood to have the potential to become any cell in the body, but the scientific reality is a bit more subtle. Different types of stem cells possess different potential outcomes. The **totipotent** stem cell, found within the inner cell mass of the blastocyst (the beginning stages of a developing embryo), has the potential to become any cell in the body. When leveraging totipotent stem cells for medical treatment, their totipotency (literally "potential for everything") can cause indeterminate differentiation problems, meaning the wrong tissue could grow in the wrong place. **Progenitor** stem cells, such as mesenchymal and hematopoietic stem cells, turn into a broad but already partly predetermined category of tissues.

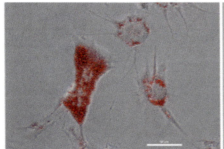
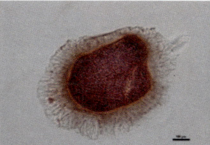
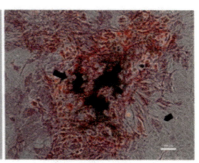

The same line of stem cells differentiated into a fat cell (left), bone cell (middle), and nerve cell (right). – Courtesy of Dr. W. Mark Erwin, University of Toronto

Further maturity gives birth to **precursor** cells that become a line of one or two tissues. Precursor cells are not quite stem cells and not quite mature cells (adult stem cells.) Finally, **mature cells** represent specific tissue.[22][23] These four cell types are not absolutely demarcated; there is some overlap in their function.

	STEM CELL HIERARCHY
Totipotent (blastocyst)	Can become any cell or any tissue
Progenitor (umbilical cord stem cells)	Can become almost any cell or tissue with a preference for certain tissue types (i.e., mostly connective tissue with some blood cells)
Precursor (adult stem cells)	Can become a cell or a tissue of a particular type (i.e., ligaments, muscles or cartilage, and not endocrine cells)
Mature (adult cells)	Fully specialized cells (i.e., muscle cells, blood cells, and so on) with no further transformative potential

How are stem cells collected?

The first step in collecting stem cells and many other regenerative products from live birth material includes retrieving the placenta, umbilical cord, and perinatal blood. For live stem cell products, birth assets are made available for later therapeutic use by creating a flowable graft. There are a few established and effective techniques to do these things. The next challenge is to stabilize the sample, analogous to stabilizing a car accident victim before transport to a hospital. Finally, the flowable graft must be cryopreserved (frozen) to minimize cell damage and death. Once properly cryopreserved, the sample can retain its regenerative potential for many years if properly stored.

Cord blood, rich with blood stem cells, can be easily made into a usable cell preparation: laboratories remove the red blood cells from the cord blood. The remaining cells may be used for transplantation through infusion or injection.

The Wharton's jelly comprising the cord wall, where most mesenchymal stem cells reside, is more difficult to turn into a clinically useful preparation. The FDA recommends that laboratories not employ enzymatic treatment (tissue liquefied by enzymes) of the umbilical cord planned for clinical use. Instead, the cord needs to be mechanically broken to be made soft and eventually flowable. This mechanical process puts additional stress on the cells and causes many of them to die.

Further, thawed blood and cord tissue may undergo the so-called "apoptotic cascade" phenomenon, when dying cells signal nearby healthy cells to die. Labs use different proprietary technologies to mitigate this attrition process, but very few do this effectively. The unfortunate result is that most live stem cell preparations on the market arrive at the doctor's office with few (if any) living cells. This attrition can occur at any step of the process, including when retrieving the raw samples, the mechanical processes to make the sample flowable, the cryopreservation process, and even the thawing and usage techniques.

For these reasons, patients have to be mindful of which supplier provides stem cells to their doctors. Presently no centralized quality control exists, and laboratories frequently present false claims about their products' viability and quality.

Stem cells manufacture and release multiple chemicals. Vesicles (small fluid-filled, lipid encased structures expelled by stem cells) contain many beneficial substances. When outside of the cell, vesicles are called exosomes. Exosomes contain parts (including proteins, DNA, RNA, etc.) of the cells that secrete them. In addition, various active ingredients may be released unpackaged, free-floating, or uncaged when stem cells fall apart. Amniotic fluid is often used to harvest such material. Collecting exosomes is a very delicate process that we will address later.

Autologous and allogeneic stem cells

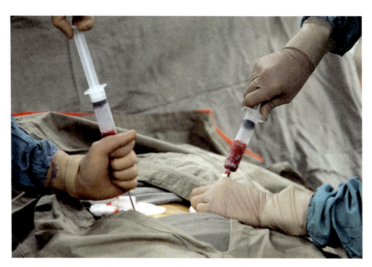
Invasive bone marrow harvesting from a patient

Autologous stem cells come from your body. They are your own cells with developed immune markers. Adult stem cells are a double-edged sword. They are as old as the donor, subject to environmental factors, fewer in number, and less potent (see "Telomeres and aging" on page 22). Adult stem cells are more precursor than progenitor cells and, as such, prefer to develop into a particular type of tissue. Consequently, when transplanted, they may experience aberrant differentiation, including tumorigenesis. In other words, experience shows that your own autologous adult stem cells can sometimes develop into cancer.

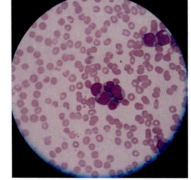
Stem cells in bone marrow

Likewise, adult stem cells collected from fat are in fat for a reason: They are more suitable for turning into fat than any other tissue. Harvesting adult stem cells from bone marrow seems better and more diverse therapeutically because of the presence of hematopoietic stem cells in addition to mesenchymal stem cells (see "Mesenchymal and hematopoietic stem cells" on page 16), but harvesting is more traumatic and expensive.[24][25]

Allogeneic stem cells come from a donor. If they come from an adult donor, they are **adult allogeneic stem cells** that have already developed immune markers and are commonly seen as foreign by the recipient immune system. This causes autoimmune rejection and the need for active immunosuppression prescribed by the treating physician.

Umbilical Cord Stem Cells	Allogeneic Adult Stem Cells	Autologous Adult Stem Cells
Have no immune markers	Have immune markers	Have immune markers
Are not rejected by the recipient's immune system	Likely to be rejected by the recipient's immune system	May be rejected by the recipient's immune system even though the cells come from their own body

Umbilical cord-derived allogeneic stem cells, on the contrary, are too young to form human leukocyte antigens (HLA), and therefore, they do not possess immune expression. The major histocompatibility complex (MHC) is not developed, making immune conflict highly unlikely with an adult host.[26] When allogeneic umbilical cord stem cells are used clinically, there is no need to test for immune compatibility or involve the patient in immunosuppression to avoid graft rejection.

MHC and HLA are created to protect our bodies from invaders. Cord stem cells are not seen as foreigners by the recipient's immune system and are not subject to attack. In other words, both autologous adult and allogeneic umbilical cord stem cells are likely safe with respect to immune compatibility, with allogeneic cells being the safest.

Mesenchymal and hematopoietic stem cells

Hematopoietic stem cells are present primarily in blood and bone marrow. They differentiate into blood cells and produce extracellular components overlapping with those secreted by mesenchymal stem cells.

Most current stem cell research is focused on mesenchymal cells. The term "**mesenchymal stem cell**" (MSC) was coined in 1991 by Dr. Arnold Caplan, but its meaning continues to evolve.[27] Since 2010, Dr. Caplan has been trying to make the abbreviation "MSC" stand for "medicinal signaling cell(s)." He explains that MSCs can be induced to differentiate in culture, but they do not easily do this in a live organism.

Mesenchymal stem cells marked with fluorescence

Mesenchyme is the embryonic connective tissue derived from the mesoderm, which differentiates into hematopoietic and connective tissue. Of note, MSCs were once thought not to differentiate into hematopoietic cells. The definition of mesenchymal stem cells has changed, as they are known to produce more tissue types than originally believed. The current definition is based on the presence or absence of specific molecules on the cell's surface and other factors. MSCs cannot be verified by visual appearance (see table below).[28]

Current Scientific Definition of Mesenchymal Stem Cells
• Are plastic-adherent when maintained in standard culture conditions
• Express the cell surface markers CD105, CD73, and CD90
• Lack expression of CD45, CD34, CD14 or CD11b, CD79 or CD19, and HLA-DR
• Differentiate to osteoblasts, adipocytes, and chondroblasts in vitro

Mesenchymal stem cells may come from anywhere in the body – not only from the umbilical cord. In this case, they are called autologous mesenchymal cells. They are primarily harvested from bone marrow and adipose (fat) tissue.[29] [30] [31] [32] The umbilical cord wall houses a particularly large mesenchymal stem cell population.

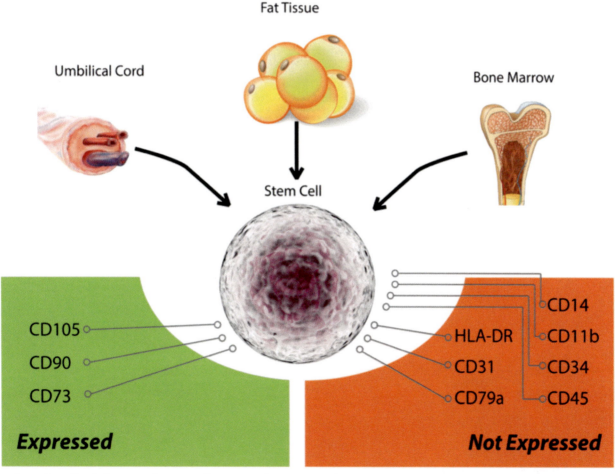

The scientific definition of stem cells comes from a set of specific factors a cell does or does not possess. It is impossible to visually identify a stem cell as it does not look any different from other cells.

Adult stem cells derived from adipose tissue will recruit other cells to be more effective within the target niche (the area needing repair.) Bone marrow stem cells are even more effective at recruiting other cells because marrow contains both hematopoietic and mesenchymal cells. Umbilical cord stem cells, by virtue of their youth, are expected to be even more potent and efficient, though this has yet to be scientifically confirmed.

All stem cell preparations contain a variety of cells. It is currently technologically impossible to have a sample with 100% mesenchymal stem cells. The difference is the proportion of cells in a sample. Hematopoietic stem cells differentiate into white and red blood cells and plasma components, which aid the immune system. Lymphocytes, monocytes, and macrophages also come out of this cell line, aiding in anti-inflammatory processes. As mentioned earlier, mesenchymal cells differentiate into connective tissue and are involved in organ repair. Hematopoietic cells do not form scaffolding, which may explain why they are, to some degree, less effective in tissue and organ repair but likely more potent in immune regulation.

Different stem cell products significantly overlap in their mechanism of action and applications. A combination of mesenchymal and hematopoietic stem cells provides the most balanced and all-encompassing influence on the body.

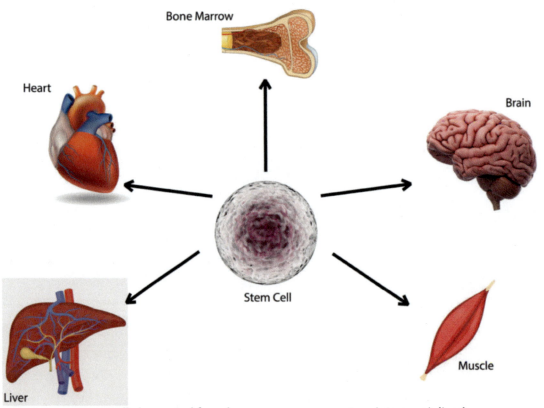

Stem cells harvested from bone marrow may mature into specialized tissue cells, depending on where the stem cells are placed.

Fetal wound healing

Newborns are, as a rule, healthier than adults. Why? Because during fetal development, active stem cells continuously repair their tissue.

In the 1980s, surgeons observed that babies were born with remarkably limited deformities after intrauterine surgeries (surgery performed on a baby before birth). Fetal healing occurs rapidly and with minimal scar formation. Therefore. using umbilical cord stem cells to treat adult wounds holds major promise.

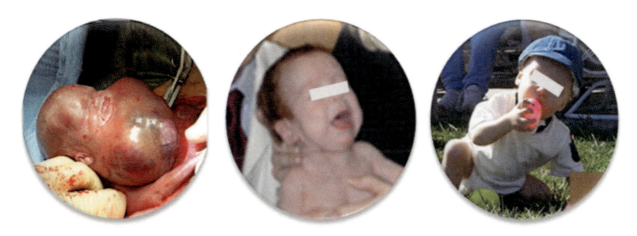

Intrauterine surgery to remove disfiguring facial tumor from a fetus (left). The same baby at birth (middle) and as a healthy toddler with minimal to no scarring (right). Courtesy Dr. Michael Harrison, Univ of California, San Francisco

In itself, the amniotic membrane is an active organ, increasing the potency of the adjacent stem cells. Seeding the amniotic membrane with umbilical cord stem cells multiplies the healing property of both.

We are made of stem cell composite, so to speak, when we enter life. As we age, the number of stem cells drops precipitously. In old age, we hardly have any. It is estimated that just one out of every two million body cells is a stem cell by age 80. Harvesting stem cells from an older donor for autologous treatment is a chore. There are fewer stem cells, and even those possess limited regenerative ability.

Amniotic and umbilical stem cell products

The birth waste of a healthy newborn provides an abundant source of stem cells. These products are not sourced from aborted fetuses. The clinical use of embryonic stem cells is strictly prohibited in the United States (see "Embryonic stem cells" on page 35).

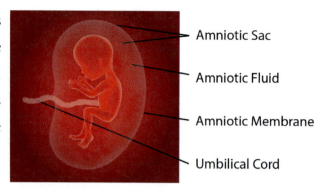

Amniotic fluid (the liquid that cushions a growing fetus) practically lacks live stem cells but is rich with cytokines and growth factors produced by stem cells. Exosomes, secreted by stem cells, may also be found in amniotic fluid. There are many amniotic fluid-derived products on the market. They have a higher concentration of active factors but produce only local time-limited connective tissue repair and do not seem to repair the immune system.[33]

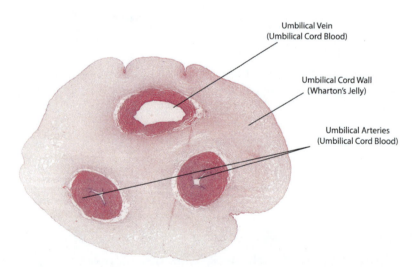

This umbilical cord cross-section shows several sources of umbilical stem cells. The vein (top) carries oxygenated umbilical cord blood from mother to embryo. The arteries (bottom left and right) carry blood from the embryo back to the placenta.

The **amniotic membrane** (the lining of the embryonic sack) is covered with stem cells. It may be used topically as a healing barrier treatment for burns, wounds, or spina bifida, to give a few examples.[34] However, understanding the practical uses of viable stem cells from the amniotic membrane will require much more investigation. Due to FDA regulatory changes in 2021, cellular products derived from amniotic fluid and amniotic membrane have become easier than live stem cells to use clinically. See "Appendix 3: Amniotic Product Components" on page 86.

Wharton's jelly (**umbilical cord wall**) cells are mostly mesenchymal cells that are especially suitable for becoming connective tissue. **Umbilical cord blood** cells are mostly hematopoietic cells that are especially suitable for becoming blood cells and immune regulators.

Umbilical cord blood and umbilical cord wall-derived products have been shown to be the most promising and safest cells for human clinical use. Because of their higher activity, it is expected that transplanted umbilical cord stem cells may increase the vitality of adult stem cells already present in the recipient's body. Both mesenchymal and hematopoietic cells are more prevalent in the umbilical cord.[35] [36]

> **Case of shoulder arthritis cure**
>
> Mr. B was recommended to have shoulder replacement surgery by his orthopedic surgeon. But, Mr. B wanted to explore his options to avoid an expensive and invasive surgical treatment with a long recovery time. He received a single injection of umbilical cord wall stem cells into his shoulder joint. His pain decreased within several days, and his range of motion improved within a week. Mr. B is pain-free with no need for surgery for over five years since his one stem cell treatment.

Furthermore, umbilical cord blood and Wharton's jelly stem cells have so far not been reported to induce neoplasia (cancer). We can estimate cancer risk by the likelihood of spontaneous cell mutations. By making stem cells immortal in a lab and allowing them to divide endlessly, a Harvard study showed that the first cancer mutation was observed after 1 million divisions, suggesting that umbilical cord blood stem cells have an extremely small likelihood of turning cancerous.[37]

	UMBILICAL CORD STEM CELLS		**ADULT STEM CELLS**		**EMBRYONIC STEM CELLS**
	Umbilical cord wall Wharton's Jelly	Umbilical cord blood	Adult autologous stem cells	Adult allogeneic stem cells	
Immune Response	?	?	+	++	+
Likely Risk of Oncogenesis	?	?	+	++	++
Composition of Cells	Mostly Mesenchymal	Mostly Hematopoietic	Mixed depending on harvest site	Mixed depending on harvest site	Mostly Mesenchymal
Risk of Uncertain Differentiation	+	+	++	+++	+++

Cellular and extracellular products

Stem cells are largely dormant within the body until activated to multiply, propagate, and influence surrounding tissues. These activities include migrating within damaged organs and healing through both physical contact and secretory function.

The migration of stem cells within the body is a complex and controversial subject, bound up with the question of how stem cells respond to damaged cells and tissues (see also "Intramuscular injections" on page 63). Stem cells may repair by their proximity to other cells, in which case they must remain in physical contact with the damaged cells, or by secreting extracellular components that spread around the body and work remotely from the stem cell. The extracellular and extra-exosomal components of stem cells (**matrix**) can be collected, preserved, and used clinically for tissue repair. The effect of matrix products is time-limited and is mostly local. The term "stem cell matrix" lacks a precise definition and usually refers to an assembly of fibrous proteins and growth factors derived from stem cells with no actual live stem cells in the composition. Matrix is not well-suited for IV infusion; instead, it is usually transplanted directly into target tissue such as a joint or muscle.

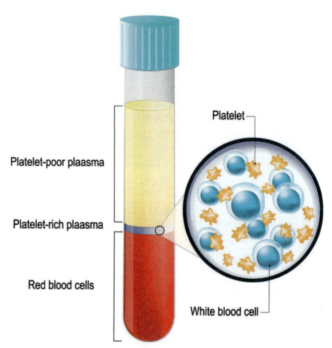

PRP is a fraction of a blood sample.

Platelet-rich plasma (PRP) is related to stem cell matrix but is not per se; it is the activated expression of a host of growth factors secreted by platelets that, in turn, act upon the tissue target, such as tendon or ligament. PRP is commonly used because it contains fairly concentrated extracellular ingredients such as growth factors, cytokines, and trophic factors, that come from adult platelets; as such, it can facilitate healing and promote the activity of the native stem cells in the surrounding tissues.[38][39][40][41] More and more studies show that PRP treatment is not objectively effective and could be placebo-related.

Consistent with previous negative reports, the Journal of the American Medical Association, at the end of November 2021, published a study of intra-articular injections of PRP to patients with symptomatic mild-to-moderate knee osteoarthritis. The study did not show significant improvement in knee pain or cartilage rebuilding compared with a placebo saline injection. The authors concluded that the study findings did not support the use of PRP for the management of knee osteoarthritis.[42]

Some see PRP as a type of prolotherapy with the potential to strengthen tissues by forming new connective tissue fibers and possibly enhancing the properties of existing ones. Like amniotic fluid-derived products, PRP does not stabilize the immune system but may produce local connective tissue repair that lasts for a limited time. Depending on the location, a positive function of PRP might be the secondary induction of stem cells located near the injection site. In other words, PRP may induce native stem cells to work better.

On the contrary, a recent paper reports that PRP delivered in vivo (to a live organism) is unlikely to activate endogenous stem cells and enhance MSC-mediated hyaline cartilage formation.[43] While the study limited its investigation to PRP's effect on cartilage formation, the findings add to the controversy surrounding various claims about the utility of PRP – which type of collagen develops, the proteins involved, and so forth. In summary, much remains to be determined about both the mechanism and the outcome of PRP treatment. This kind of therapy does involve significant inflammation and the potential of undesirable long-term consequences of scarring. Despite shaky scientific ground, PRP is widely used, and many patients report clinical benefits. As it happens, we know that "something is there"; we just do not know how to explain it.

PRP may be made from umbilical cord blood as well as the patient's own blood. Donors with hormonal challenges, morbidities, and post-menopausal women are thought to have less stimulatory PRP.

One study found that adding even 0.1% of umbilical cord PRP to autologous adult PRP produces a disproportionate, many-fold increase in potency, which testifies to the higher biological activity of young tissue versus mature tissue.[44] The umbilical cord cytokine concentration far exceeds that of an adult PRP. Some factors appear to be absent from PRP. This may explain, in part, the higher therapeutic potency of live stem cell treatment.

Although one must be wary of drawing far-reaching conclusions from a single study, it makes intuitive sense that the vigor of youth would enhance stem cell products.

Usually, cellular products refer to the preparations of live stem cells. The goal of such preparations is to utilize a full unobstructed force of nature with the idea to let stem cells do what they are created to do: build up and repair the human body.

A subgroup of cellular products consists of whole cells collected from birth waste that are not guaranteed to be alive. Such cells are usually preserved with a higher DMSO concentration, which makes intravenous administration contraindicated. Such products are limited to peripheral use for joint and soft tissue implantation. Regenative Labs and other companies offer such biologics to the marketplace.

The third major group of regenerative products is exosomes. They are packages of growth factors and cytokines expelled from the cells. Exosomal products are the latest addition to the market. They are easier to study and preserve than live cells; this makes them cheaper and possibly safer to use.

Telomeres and aging

Telomeres are the caps on the ends of chromosomes that prevent the chromosomes from fraying or falling apart. Without those caps, chromosomes are unstable. Uncapped chromosomes unwind and disintegrate, or fuse with adjacent chromosomes, causing cell death.

Every time cells divide, the telomeres shorten; this is why we age and why our tissues get older.[45] We are born with about eight thousand base telomeres and have ten times fewer when we die from old age.

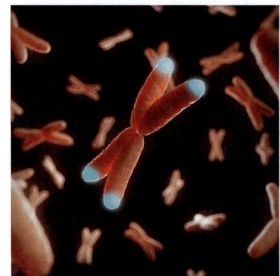
Telomeres are depicted here as blue caps on the ends of the chromosomal arms.

Umbilical cord stem cells have the maximum length telomeres. When they reproduce and repair adult tissue, they donate younger chromosomes, rejuvenating adult tissue.[46] [47] This is a source of optimism for regenerative medicine: With regular stem cell treatment, the body is not only rejuvenated – it likely ages slower.

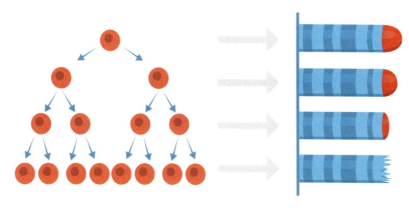

Telomeres shorten with each cell division.

Adult tissue stem cells have short telomeres; as such, they may be active for repair but not for rejuvenation – but of course, old stem cells with shorter telomeres are still better than fully matured adult cells.[48]

Aging stem cells enter a state called "**senescence**." Such cells retain stem cell function but stop dividing. By mid-age, most stem cells lose the ability to divide, although they continue to repair; this is why the number of stem cells dwindles, and aging accelerates.[49][50] This is another reason adult stem cells cannot fully compete with umbilical cord stem cells.

Aging stem cells also suffer from mitochondrial dysfunction, which means the cell powerhouses – mitochondria – work less and less efficiently as we age. Umbilical cord stem cells normally do not share that problem.

> Case of ileitis cure:
>
> Mr. C had explored doing stem cell treatment for general health reasons. When he came to the appointment to receive an infusion of mixed blood/cord stem cells, his current condition was worrisome. The evening before, he had developed abdominal pain and nausea, and by the time of the appointment, he was sitting bent over, complaining of great discomfort. A surgeon saw Mr. C immediately, appendicitis was suspected, and an abdominal CT ordered. His CT scans showed a severely inflamed and swollen intestinal tract, indicative of ileitis or Crohn's Disease. We proceeded with the scheduled stem cell infusion as it was known to be anti-inflammatory and potentially helpful for Crohn's Disease.
>
> Mr. C's pain decreased dramatically within several hours, and all symptoms disappeared by the next morning, using no medications of any kind. The abdominal CT was repeated in ten days and showed completely normal small and large intestines. Mr. C remains healthy ever since.

In a lab setting, stem cells have been observed to divide approximately every 28 hours and about 70 times. This division cannot be reliably shown in a live organism. The replication rate is variable between species. In humans, multiplication is reported to be as fast as a few hours and as slow as every 40 weeks, and this is why the original infused cells theoretically may be present in the body for up to three to six months or more. Unlike adult tissue, which has been exposed to radiation, toxins, and mutations, the DNA of umbilical stem cells is young and transposes these features onto the host in which they find a new life.

However, the long-term preservation of whole umbilical cord or cord blood may be technically difficult, and there is no guarantee that cells survive the process (see "Vitality and preservation" on page 45). Also, many years of paying for storage may not be cost-effective.

Estimating the number of cells

Claims of a specific number of cells in a preparation are usually misleading if not completely fraudulent. Patients and physicians need to pay special attention to claims of high cell counts. A reported and marketed number of cells per volume is likely just that: marketing. A high number of live cells within a given volume (per 1 cc or 1 ml, for example) is difficult to impossible to achieve biologically. Stem cells die due to crowding, and then the apoptotic cascade (see "How are stem cells collected?" on page 14) finishes most of the rest of them. It is reasonable to understand that more than 10 million live stem cells per 1cc is currently technologically unlikely.

It is also crucial to be aware of the different levels of quality available. Viability is more important for live cell products than the cell count number. Again: the reputation, ethics, and scientific standing of the lab are the keys to trusting the stem cell products you use.

It is not scientific but a simple, practical hint to judging flowable products: if the vial content is colorless and/or clear, it is likely a poor-quality sample and should not be trusted. Cells will contribute to turbidity; plasma will impart a distinct amber hue. The absence of color and opacity indicates a lack of cells and plasma in the preparation – whereas a clear, translucent sample in most cases is primarily saline. This rule doesnt apply to acellular products, because cells are not present in their composition.

Exosomes

All tissue cells, including stem cells, produce exosomes, packaged payloads of growth factors, cytokines, and other factors destined for secretion from the cell. Nearly all good stem cell preparations will be a primitive source of exosomes in varying degrees of health and integrity.

> **Asthma symptom control:**
>
> Ms. D traveled from California along with her friend, who was a current stem cell patient in our clinic. Ms. D had an almost non-stop asthmatic cough that disabled her to the point that she could not do her job. Her condition was obviously associated with an oak allergy, as these trees surrounded her home. Seeing improvement in her friend's conditions, Ms. D decided to try treatments herself. Umbilical cord blood stem cells almost immediately stopped her cough and improved her breathing.
>
> She flew home feeling well. Her improvement lasted for several months despite her continued exposure to allergens in her environment. Since that time, she has undergone several follow-up treatments with the same results, immediate improvement with a slow return of the symptoms after going back home. For her long-term benefit, Ms. D would be wise to move away from the allergens and other environmental factors that continue to undermine her health.

Exosomes are one of the many components of cellular life – and a relatively simple one. A cell is encircled by a phospholipid cell wall surrounding multiple intracellular organs such as mitochondria, ribosomes, and other structures and features. Exosomes are cellular sub-compartments of a living cell. The Latin "exo" means "outside," so exosomes are defined by their journeys outside of the cell into the outer space of biology for signaling, consumption, or waste disposal. Other similar cellular compartments never leave the cell and are more or less distinguished along functional lines, such as vesicles, lysosomes, etc.

Like satellites, exosomes can deliver signals to surrounding cells and tissues. These signals are like a bullhorn that calls the rest of the micro-universe to attention – to march, fire, farm, or die. Some direct downstream events are amplified, and amplification, likely, is the purpose of these signals.

Exosomes can also be secreted with raw materials or "food" to benefit a greater layer: a tissue, an organ, an organism. As for waste disposal, some exosomes are garbage trucks, without which we would suffocate in our own waste. What if exosome functions could be controlled? What if the contents of the exosomes could be engineered to contain signals, designed to be amplified and have a positive effect? It would be an extraordinary tool for regenerative medicine. Likewise, it would be exciting to farm some of the most biologically active molecules in our physiology.

This exosome frontier is exciting and is begging for more exploration. The key to the future of exosomes will be how well we explore them, how little we stumble in the process, and how we deliver them to patients. Currently, we have more work to do; rigorous analysis of secreted molecules, understanding of what they do, and strict parameters to create repeatable "crops."

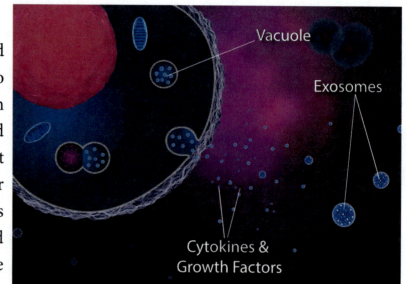

Vacuoles become exosomes when they empty their contents into the extracellular environment.

Depending on the stimulus and harvest protocols, exosomes also introduce the possibility of an unbalanced and unregulated overdose of "waste" molecules that can lead to teratogenesis or other unwanted adverse effects. This reaffirms the need to understand further all the aspects of exosome manufacture. As mentioned earlier, exosomes can come from any cells; this means they also come from cancer cells; you can guess that such exosomes would not carry healthy signals. For this reason, the source material for exosomes must be carefully selected to creat a viable therapeutic preparation. (see "Appendix 4A: Growth Regulating Factors" on page 87 and "Appendix 4B: Immune Regulating Factors" on page 88).

The term "exosomes" became a popular marketing slogan. It sounds intriguing and scientific; it carries a mysterious meaning, though, in plain English, it just means "cell secretion." In summary, "exosomes" are packaged cell secretions that can be divided into three categories:

- Waste, that is naturally thrown out of the cells (contaminants); these are the harmful exosomes.

- Negative regulating/signaling molecules, carrying messages to slow or kill certain distant cells or their function; this can be good ("kill sick cells") or bad ("kill healthy cells").

- Positive regulating/signaling molecules, carrying messages to heal, repair or improve the health and function of certain distant cells.

All three types are produced by the same cells, but only the third type of exosome is truly healthy. As mentioned above, we have not had the technology to separate those types of molecules, and, as a result, "exosome" products have been a mixture of food and trash.

In an exciting new development, the Mayo Clinic has patented a way to separate exosomes by size and chemical composition with the promise of soon bringing an approved exosome-based medication to the market. Some labs also claim an ability to presort exosomes, extracting only healthy ones through so-called nanosite technology.[51] These products are not live cells but a biologic secretions category, making them easier and cheaper to research and use clinically.

Many thousands of active molecules are produced and secreted by stem cells. Each has a specific purpose, poorly known or completely unknown to us, which is unfortunate. What is exciting is that when we do research them, one by one, we'll have incredible tools to specifically regulate everything in our bodies. Even more appealing is the potential ability to artificially synthesize specific molecules for a specific purpose in an individual patient. When we learn enough from stem cells, we will no longer need to harvest them.

Understandably, human research is complicated. Studying live processes in the body is frequently too risky; this applies to stem cells and exosomes. A novel approach to circumvent this challenge is being developed: avatar mice. The avatar system allows the production of mice that mirror human tissue, including the manufacture of exosomes. This allows studying down to a molecular level what happens with the synthesis, composition, secretion, distribution, and function of exosomes. Such studies will let us know what works – a cell, an exosome, or a specific cytokine. This extensive work requires scientific rigor and expertise, affordable only to a few places. The Mayo Clinic is one such place, pioneering exosome research.

It is not sufficient to call a cell secretion "an exosome." What exosome is has to be specifically defined; only then can researchers compare apples to apples. Consider an adult human defined by size (say between two and 8 feet), the presence of a heart and head, and the absence of wings. A five-inch or ten feet tall winged creature is unlikely a human. The same principle applies to exosomes. With exosomes, size matters – they are usually between 50 and 150 micrometers in size, and they have specific surface markers and other markers they must not have.

I mentioned that exosomes could come from any cell, so specific sources of exosomes must be used to study them appropriately. Mesenchymal stem cells are probably the best origin of healthy exosomes, but this needs to be proven and not assumed. What is the potency, and what is the purity of exosomes? Would umbilical cord blood or cord wall cells be better sources? Would exosomes from immune cells be better for autoimmune diseases and exosomes from Warton jelly more suitable for connective tissue repair? We have more questions than answers now, but knowing what to ask is a start.

If you wonder what the contents of an exosome are, the answer is simple: anything. Millions of types of exosomes cannot be piled up with the hope that something works. Coming out with a medication-grade exosome product will require establishing set parameters for purity, potency, and allowed impurities. And then comes the question of dosing: common sense may suggest that concentration matters, but it is how to know the right dose. And last but not least: should dosing be different for different conditions?

Technically it is difficult to make dry and still active exosome products as exosomes want to stay in a solution. What to bind them with to extract from solution? How to not destroy them in the process? How to make the end product cheap enough to be available around the world? How to make storage and distribution affordable? With all these requirements, how to make it commercially viable?

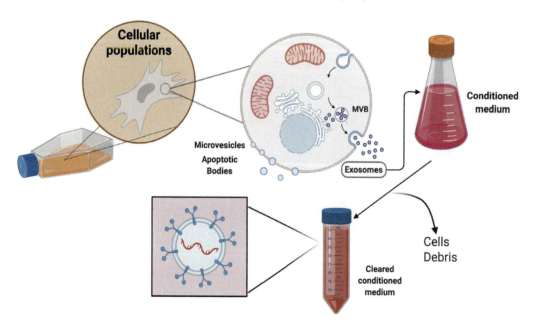

Processing of exosomes - Courtesy Atta Behfar, MD, PhD, MAYO Clinic, 2022.

The complexity of the exosome subject is staggering, but anything new seems incomprehensible in the beginning. Exosomes go beyond stem cells; they are beyond the field of regenerative medicine. Exosomes are openings into a new type of pharmacology with the potential to change the way both cytokines and medications are packaged and delivered through the body.

ANIMAL STEM CELL PRODUCTS

Stem cell research and treatment did not start with human subjects. It started with animals, whose sacrifices led to medical developments and discoveries. The use of stem cells in veterinary medicine is irreplaceable and ever-evolving. Much of the knowledge we gained in regenerative medicine, including stem cells, comes from animal research, utilizing veterinary facilities and animal laboratories. It is not wise to translate animal studies directly to humans, but they provide the building blocks of our medical knowledge.

In principle, stem cell use in animals parallels human use. Horses, cats, and dogs may benefit from stem cell treatment based on the same principles as their human friends. Treatment of the musculoskeletal system is the most common, but other applications have also been explored.[52] As in humans, both autologous and allogeneic stem cells are used. Bone marrow, fat, and blood-derived stem cell use is reported.[53][54][55][56][57] The key is not to implant stem cell material cross-species. Remember: umbilical cord stem cells from horses are good for horses, not cats. And, of course, animal stem cells are unacceptable for human use.

One of the major barriers to harvesting stem cells in animals is that umbilical cord stem cells are usually collected via c-section, which for obvious reasons, is not the normal delivery method for animals.

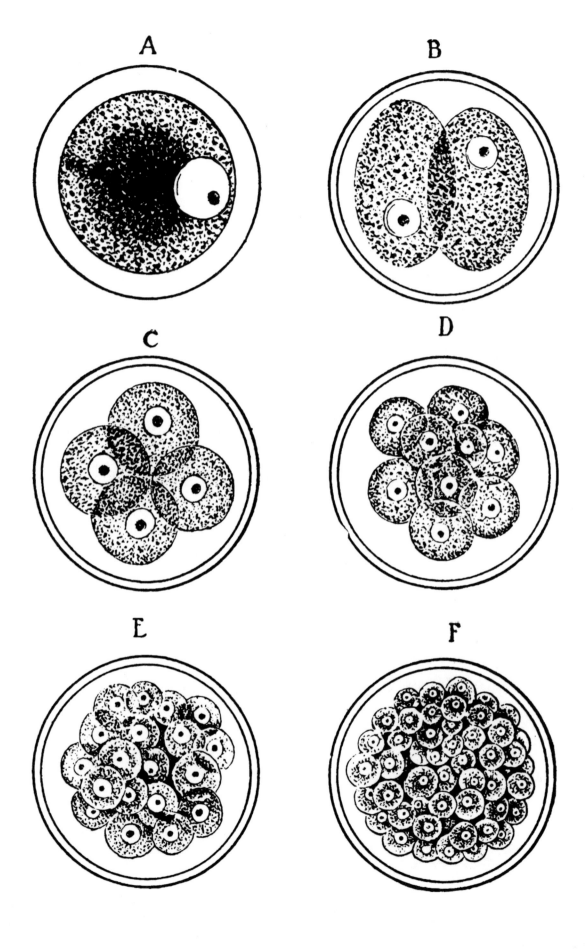

PART TWO:

PROBLEMS & CONCERNS

Stem cell problems and concerns

Before regenerative and stem cell treatments are widely adopted, many challenges must be overcome. These include regulation, harvesting, concentrating, preserving, testing for diseases, increasing survivability, etc. Gaining the required know-how is expensive and time-consuming. But the reward is great: a novel therapeutic tool that may better countless lives.

Risks of stem cell treatment

Many patients, especially the devout, will approach stem cell treatment with a false preconception about how stem cells are harvested; this is a basic complication that can be averted through education: *Embryos are not used to harvest stem cells in the United States.* The same cannot be said for some other countries.

Clinically, as with any treatment, other possible complications must always be carefully considered. Stem cell DNA may mutate in the lab when the sample is processed, or there may be an immune reaction or disease transmission. Once cells are administered, they may experience aberrant differentiation, which can cause tumors. Finally, most stem cell treatments are expensive and of unproven efficacy at this time.[58][59] Exosomes are safer from a genetic standpoint, and specific cytokines and growth factors are likely even more safe. However, as with stem cells, it is known that exosomes and other products sourced from adult tissue have expressed histocompatibility, making them visible to the recipient's immune system, thus requiring prophylactic antirejection treatments. The potential dangers of exosomes and their components are largely unknown and require more research. Recognizing the potential harm from stem cells and other biologics, governments regulate the regenerative field more and more closely.

Religious concerns

Stem cell therapy has been viewed negatively by those who feel it is immoral and against God's will. Many do not understand the stem cells used for therapy come from either excess birth material or the patients themselves. *Stem cells used for human treatment in the United States DO NOT come from fetuses or embryos.*

The big question is whether humans were meant to harness the miraculous ability of stem cells to treat pain, wounds, and other medical conditions. Ask yourself how God works. Do miracles suddenly appear from thin air? Or might we see God's hand in the miracles, large and small, produced by scientists, doctors, engineers, and even random strangers? Cutting-edge research, out-of-the-box theories, and viewing life's elements from a different angle are all random acts of kindness that have effectively led to miracles for countless people.

In today's world of medicine, regenerative therapies are both biological miracles and acts of kindness to those suffering from ailments that are not easily treated. Miracles are a choice, and they tend to take effort. The doctors, scientists, and other contributors to the developing these therapies have done so to help those suffering, and their efforts have paid off with what seems to be an effective treatment. It would be immoral to refuse these therapies for patients.

Unlike stem cells, more fundamental blocks of biological products may come from specifically bred animals or be synthesized from scratch in a lab. We are not there yet, but developments like these may eliminate religious concerns.

Embryonic stem cells

At the dawn of stem cell research, some allogeneic stem cells were derived from aborted embryos. These **embryonic stem cells** (ESCs) were the source of serious moral, ethical, and religious concerns. Clinically, embryonic stem cells also proved unreliable, and outcomes were plagued with complications. Due to the complexities in their genetic composition and state of development, transplanted embryonic cells frequently homed into the wrong area of the body. They also suffered from uncertain differentiation, maturing into unwanted tissue, including cancer.

The use of animal-derived stem cells was also clinically problematic due to the dangers of cross-species tissue transplantation. These uncertainties and unknowns led to regulatory concerns and a change in public opinion, which lead to a drastic reduction in the clinical use of stem cells in Europe and, more recently, the United States.

Due to media sensationalism, many still associate present-day stem cell treatment with ESCs. To repeat: *No human or animal ESCs are permitted for clinical use in the United States.*

Umbilical cord stem cells

In the United States, vendors of umbilical cord products collect stem cells from the donated birth waste of healthy live newborns delivered by C-section to avoid contamination. We already know that, by definition, embryonic stem cells originate from developing fetal tissue. On the other hand, umbilical cord-derived stem cells (UCSCs) are undifferentiated (meaning undeveloped). UCSCs to date have not been associated with oncogenesis (they do not cause healthy cells to turn into cancer cells), nor are they themselves known to turn into cancer. However unlikely, this negative outcome is still possible.

Furthermore, harvesting from the umbilical cord sidesteps the ethical and religious concerns associated with embryonic stem cells. The improved clinical outcomes and lack of moral hazards have made umbilical cord stem cells popular for research and clinical applications. Nonetheless, a great deal more study of the potential use of UCSCs is necessary, and present-day clinical use is entirely investigational.

Induced pluripotent stem cells

Shinya Yamanaka and John Gurdon poineered induced pluripotent stem cells (iPSC). In 2006, they showed that introducing four specific genes may turn somatic cells (such as skin or even renal epithelial cells in urine) into pluripotent stem cells. They were awarded the 2012 Nobel Prize "for the discovery that mature cells can be reprogrammed to become pluripotent."[60]

iPSCs can be derived directly from adult tissues; they bypass the need for birth material and can be made from the donor herself.[61] Such cells cannot be used in clinical medicine in the United States because of questionable safety profiles, causing tumors.[62] Their efficacy is very poor (0.01–0.1% in the original mouse study), and in addition to tumorigenicity, a genomic insertion and incomplete reprogramming further complicate iPSC use.

At the same time, they have found a prominent place in the research and development of new medications and treatments, including in psychiatry.[63] With sufficient scientific advances, iPSCs have a bright future.

Overseas stem cell treatment

Many Americans travel abroad for stem cell treatment, trusting in fantastical claims about what can optimistically be described as questionable stem cell products. You will never quite know what you are getting. In some countries, stem cells may be manipulated and grown in a medium, a process that may influence their identity (phenotype) such that they are no longer stem cells, but fibroblasts, for instance. As a result, out of a claimed 100 million cells, only a few thousand may actually be stem cells (see also "Donor and tissue screening" on page 44).

Good treatments and good products are available in the US, where regenerative products are heavily regulated for the sake of public safety. Just about everything, from harvesting and testing to preservation and distribution, is under scrutiny. This is done for the safety of the donors and patients. Laboratory and physician accountability in this country is higher than practically anywhere else. Also, restrictions on animal and embryonic stem cells relieve the original ethical concerns.

The US prohibition on cell manipulation, expansion (growing in a lab), and enhancement for clinical use adds another protection level. Stem cell expansion outside of the body, an unregulated practice at many overseas stem cell tourism destinations, increases the risk of tumorigenesis. That bears repeating: *Many stem cell tourism destinations do not regulate stem cell manipulation, which poses a higher cancer and contamination risk for patients.* Presently, the danger of stem cell expansion and enhancement is just one more reason to seek the most naive and least expanded product possible to administer to patients.[64] Future research will undoubtedly bring more knowledge for safe and beneficial stem cell expansion and manipulation. We are moving in that direction but are not there yet.

The cost of care, as well, remains an issue. Regenerative treatments are expensive due to the sophisticated process of bringing biological materials from the donor to the patient. Repeated treatments are also usually required, especially for complex conditions. The prospect of one regenerative treatment curing a chronic illness is highly unlikely and any travel abroad for such a miraculous treatment would likely end in disappointment. Safer and more affordable alternatives are available for patients seeking treatment in the United States.

There are ethical and professional clinics worldwide where reputable physicians and scientists do their best to provide the safest and most effective treatment for patients. The key for patients is to do careful research and compare clinics and doctors. One old and relevant wisdom states that "if something seems too good, it is probably not." Be very careful believing excessive and unbalanced promises.

Unfortunately, regardless of cautionary tales, the latest FDA enforcement will effectively move live stem cell clinical use and many practical innovations from the United States to foreign lands for the foreseeable future.

> **Knee arthritis cases:**
>
> Many patients in our clinic have had stem cell treatment for knee osteoarthritis, including one of our own doctors. The majority have improved enough to avoid knee replacement surgeries, had complete or almost complete pain control, and restored function for a long time. A temporary increase in local pain is common after introducing stem cells inside the joint and is directly associated with the severity of knee inflammation. This initial pain goes away, and the knee heals, but wear and tear continues, so the need for repeated treatments every three, six, or 12 months is common.

REGULATION

Responsible FDA-regulated vendors of umbilical cord products collect their biomaterials directly from the donated birth waste of healthy live newborns, making these products both ethical and practical.

Stem cell research was never banned in the US, but restrictions on funding were put in place during the George W. Bush administration. The stance was softened when President Bush signed into law the Stem Cell Therapeutic and Research Act of 2005, which provided $265 million for adult stem cell therapy, umbilical cord blood, and bone marrow treatment, and authorized $79 million for the collection of cord blood. In 2009, President Obama lifted restrictions on federal funding for stem cell research.

Bone marrow-derived stem cells have been used to treat leukemia and lymphoma for decades and this treatment is a covered benefit under some insurance policies. The FDA has approved several hematopoietic stem cell products derived from umbilical cord blood for the treatment of blood and immunological diseases.[65] However, stem cell treatments remain experimental and investigational for most health conditions – and even illegal under certain circumstances.

Several laboratories offered live stem cells and other regenerative products to medical providers. Thanks to growing availability and reliability of supply, live stem cells were part of the clinical arsenal for several years. When incorporated into an overall patient care plan, this treatment opened new horizons in medicine, allowing for more effective treatments. Nevertheless, none of these applications were without limitations.

Through May of 2021, biological products such as stem cells were defined in subsection 361, section 1271, title 21 of the code of federal regulations. This assignment allowed stem cells to be studied either under Institutional Review Board (IRB) guidance (which requires formal steps in research and investigation of new treatments) or under an investigator-guided study format (which is very broad and much less formal). As a result, stem cells were used in a clinical setting without rigorous regulation. This could be risky from a safety standpoint but allows for significant innovation and exploration of clinical applications.

The whole regenerative medicine field drastically changed in 2021. Currently, many biologics derived from birth waste, including live stem cells, are regulated under subsection 351 instead of 361. The difference is that 351 regulates the development of medications. As of now, complex-content biologics are equated to single-molecule medications in the way they have to be proven safe and effective. This must be government-approved under an Investigational New Drug (IND) application. The barrier to receiving official IND status is high, expensive, and narrow. Each application covers only specific treatments of a specific site. For instance, stem cell IND for treatment of knee osteoarthritis would not cover shoulder treatment and vice versa. The expense and time requirements of such studies are prohibitive. We'll come back to regulatory issues later in the book.

In addition to INDs, companies that produce, clean, test, and distribute these biologics adhere to multiple protocols established by specialty companies, tissue banks, blood banks, the FDA, and the Center for Biological Evaluation and Research.[66]

As I just mentioned, the logistics of the regenerative medicine industry sharply changed in June 2021, when the FDA implemented its latest regulations limiting the clinical use of stem cells and related products. It starts with strict regulations on the marketing of biologic therapies, which have been coming for a long time. For example, in May 2019, the Food and Drug Administration (FDA) warned a Scottsdale, Arizona, company that it might be subject to prosecution for marketing unapproved stem cell products to treat various diseases and conditions. The acting FDA Commissioner said: "We continue to see companies and individuals use questionable marketing campaigns to take advantage of vulnerable patients and their families with unproven claims about their unapproved stem cell products." [67] In August 2020, the FDA issued a warning letter to another stem cell vendor regarding "Unapproved and Misbranded Product Related to Coronavirus Disease 2019 (COVID-19)." [68]

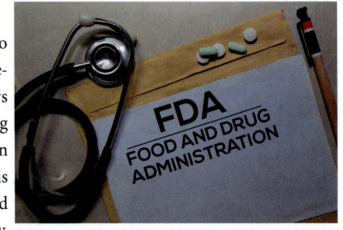

Back in 2017, the FDA issued guidance to human cells, tissues, and cellular and tissue-based product (HCT/P) manufacturers and healthcare providers regarding biologic products covered under section 361 of the PHS Act (42 U.S.C. 264). This essentially impacted all of the stem cell and regenerative medicine suppliers. Ultimately, this guidance became regulation, and the FDA published a period of enforcement discretion, which extended through May 31, 2021. As of June 1, 2021, the FDA considers most if not all products previously approved for human use as ineligible for section 361. The FDA published a Patient and Consumer Information release to inform the public about these changes on June 3, 2021.[69] The previous practice of allowing the use of stem cells for clinical research has been limited to only stem cell products approved by the FDA under investigational new drug applications (INDs). Under these new rules, most stem cells and related products must go through the same approval process as new medications. This extremely expensive and lengthy process is likely only affordable for large institutions and pharmaceutical companies. Manufacturing and shipping live stem cell products are now nearly impossible in the United States. As of the end of 2021, the availability of live stem cell products is effectively zero. As frequently happens in government, good intentions to assure product safety, ethical marketing, and clinical benefits turn into prohibition and over-regulation, invariably slowing scientific progress.

It is impossible to study live cells with tens to hundreds of thousands of active molecules, the same way a single molecule medication is investigated. As a result, most of the industry pivoted to study specific cytokines, growth factors, and exosomes. This real science will undoubtedly bring exciting discoveries but will likely take dozens of years and billions of dollars. Ultimately, it is akin to allowing studies of hearts or livers but not allowing studies of the whole organism. Instead of building roads, the government creates roadblocks, "kill the baby to protect the baby." Live stem cells and the ingredients they manufacture are not the same. Clinical trials are needed to improve the efficacy and safety of all products and treatments. Undoubtedly, the rules will change in the future, but for now, patients go underground or seek completely unregulated treatments elsewhere around the world. This will cause more problems than appropriately regulated and measured treatments inside the United States. The saddest part is that these prohibitions have been broadly applied to regenerative medicine treatments, not just stem cells.

FDA issued a detailed document titled Regulatory Considerations for Human Cells, Tissues, and Cellular and Tissue-Based Products: Minimal Manipulation and Homologous Use Guidance for Industry and Food and Drug Administration Staff which explains details of the FDA requirements for such products. The actual text of recommendations may be found at https://www.fda.gov/vaccines-blood-biologics/guidance-compliance-regulatory-information-biologics/biologics-guidances and https://www.fda.gov/CombinationProducts/default.htm

It boils down to the FDA frowning on the term "stem cell" or claims of systemic action. Products that have avoided re-classification to section 351 (drug) have embraced terms like "regenerative biologics" and focus on local homologous action. The FDA provides a flowchart to help clarify the distinctions between Sections 351 and 361, see "Appendix 5: Section 351 vs. 361 Flowchart" on page 89.

What is prohibited?

Cross-species animal stem cell treatment is not recommended, and human embryonic stem cells are not permitted for clinical use. At the time of writing, the FDA does not allow, for clinical use, any modification of stem cells, such as outside-the-body expansion (multiplying stem cells in a laboratory) or sorting (separating different cells based on some parameter). The idea of making stem cells somehow better through scientific manipulation holds promise and likely will become a clinical reality in the future. But for now, as already mentioned, this is only performed in a laboratory setting, primarily overseas.

In August 2017, the FDA took action against a California company for mixing stem cells with viruses, with the idea of injecting the mixture into tumors of cancer patients.[70] The idea of having stem cells activating viruses and working together makes sense. However, such stem cell use is currently not allowed in clinical practice due to unacceptable risk and lack of safety data. Currently, no manipulation of stem cells is permitted. However, newer clinical trials have selected a certain class of stem cells for use, such as several Mesoblast trials.[71] With sufficient research, stem cell manipulation may be more accepted and even surpass unaltered stem cell efficacy. The time for this practice has is yet to come.

Meanwhile, as mentioned earlier, the FDA limits stem cells, exosomes, amniotic fluid, and orthobiologics to uses defined within an IND. It is not the FDA's goal to stop the use of biologic products, but confusion about what is allowed and under what circumstances persists. It will take time for the dust of change to settle and the cloud of what can be done outside of approved clinical trials established.

Donating stem cells & to whom they belong

There are many social questions surrounding stem cell donations. Some have answers, and others do not. Federal guidelines outline what happens when a mother wants to preserve her newborn's umbilical cord stem cells. These guidelines regulate the collection, processing, testing, banking, packaging, and distribution of stem cells.[72]

Suppose new parents collect and preserve a newborn's umbilical cord stem cells at birth. Can parents or another relative use the baby's preserved cells? The FDA allows the use of stem cells in first and second-degree relatives, but this practice is ethically questionable.[73] Only when stem cells come from the adult recipient themself, is there no question of ownership; adult autologous cells belong to the donor.

Allogeneic stem cell samples are a more complicated issue. Other than discarding it as waste, a pregnant mother has very few options for their new baby's cord material: she can pay to have it banked with a private cord bank (basically storing her property) or donate it to a private or public cord bank. All of these have different ramifications. Otherwise, birth waste has historically been a burden and is routinely incinerated or discarded with associated expenses.

When the parent chooses to bank their child's cord material privately, they are making a significant financial investment for a long time. About one in 5,000 banked samples is used; most are never claimed. In these cases, the mother's body produces the placenta and umbilical cord with all their contents before the sample goes to the cord blood bank. Does this mean that the mother owns stem cells? Presently this is how government regulators see it. Until the child reaches 18 years of age, the mother can decide how to use the cells. What if the baby's parents are divorced, and the child's father wants to use stem cells for himself or a child from another marriage? Does he have equal rights with the mother? Due to stem cell regulation changes in the United States, there is now a paradoxical situation where you can store your own stem cells but not use them, as medical providers are limited in how these materials can be used outside of a formal research protocol. This situation is likely temporary until regulations are amended.

Biologically and genetically, stem cells develop from an embryo and technically represent the baby's tissue. I mentioned an ethical dilemma in an earlier part of this book: if stem cells from the baby are used on another person before the child is 18 years old, is it fair to the child who herself may need the cells for future treatment? Would a mother potentially have another baby to harvest stem cells for a different, sick child? Such ethical questions do not yet have a clear answer. I believe that ethical pitfalls may be avoided if privately collected stem cells were seen as belonging to the child, and using the cells for the benefit of someone else would not be acceptable.

With all that, life is complicated. What if a child's sibling is ill and only stem cell treatment offers a reasonable solution? What is more ethical – to keep stem cells for the future needs of a child they belong to or potentially save a sibling's life? What about saving a parent's

---

Chronic Obstructive Pulmonary Disease (COPD) improvement:

COPD is a common comorbid condition in our patients. When patients are treated with intravenous stem cells, we see improvements in both the target disease and in lung function. Patients regularly report that they stop using oxygen, breathe better, need fewer or no inhalers, and perform tasks without losing breath. This improvement rarely lasts for more than six months and frequently requires repeated treatment to sustain it. Nevertheless, their breathing improves so much that patients regularly choose to come back for booster infusions.

life? We do not have answers to these questions, and the courts will eventually decide some, if not most, of these issues.

If the mother chooses to donate her child's cord material to a public cord blood bank, the ownership issue is easy; the stem cells belong to the bank because it is all done at their expense. However, this process has proven to be very expensive. In this case, the donated cells have to undergo HLA typing for compatibility with a recipient (especially if the bone marrow is collected). Due to the complexities, the price is high and the demand is low – making it unaffordable for both the bank and the patient. This is sending many public stem cell banks out of business.

The mother's third but likely most practical and economical choice is to donate their child's birth material to a private cord blood bank. Again, the material, once donated, belongs to the blood bank. The processing and storage costs are covered by the sale of the products created from the donated material. Clinics that use these stem cell products need to be careful to source them from a reliable lab or cord bank. Patients seeking stem cell treatments should be informed about these product sources.

DONOR AND TISSUE SCREENING

Donating umbilical cord tissue is voluntary and free. The mother has to be mentally capable of making decisions. Family screening, viral, bacterial, and immunologic screenings are all done. The cells cannot be modified, induced, expanded, enhanced, or altered in a clinical setting. In the United States, animal mediums (including bovine serum) cannot be legally used in clinical practice to multiply cells outside of the mother's body.

Examples of Donor Screening
Competency screening
Parental social screening
Viral and bacterial infectious disease screening
Genetic screening
Tryptic Soy Agar sterility test on both mother and cord blood to test for diseases and abnormalities

TESTING AND COUNTING CELLS

Testing is automated and allows for analyzing the content of growth factors, cytokines, mutations, RNA, DNA, and the proportion of live and dead cells. Umbilical cord blood contains hundreds of thousands to millions of stem cells depending on the donor. Wharton's jelly contains even more cells, but it would be a mistake to think that all those cells are stem cells or mesenchymal stem cells, for that matter.

Counting stem cells in a blood/tissue sample is a daunting process. The difference between cell types is not obvious, and they cannot be easily identified. The number of stem cells in a sample is only a rough approximation. One would be wise to turn a skeptical eye to any company's claims on a cell count for their product. A reputable vendor should perform appropriate cell selection such as FACS/cell sorting with appropriate markers and control. Since the COVID pandemic, it may not be safe to harvest birth waste material, so labs try to use pre-COVID samples as much as possible

Examples of Umbilical Cord Tissue Testing
Cytomegalovirus IgG and IgM
West Nile Virus Nucleic Acid Test
Zika Virus PCR test and IgM
Human T-lymphotropic virus I and II antibodies
HIV Type I and II and O antibodies
RPR (nontreponemal)
CAPITA (treponemal)
Hep. B antibody, antigen, and nucleic acid test
Hep. C antibodies and Nucleic Acid Test
COVID-19

Recently collaborative research at the Universities of Maryland, Pennsylvania, and Emory University developed a new technology called "liquid biopsy" that monitors stem cells by analyses of exosomes secreted by the transplanted cells. According to Dr. Kaushal of the University of Maryland, various proteins, nucleic acids, and micro ribonucleic acids are sorted to determine whether stem cell therapy will be effective for an individual patient. It was found that the contents of the exosomes in live organisms differed substantially from what they had produced in the lab, indicating the cells changed after transplantation.[74] This process still does not determine how many cells were transplanted but allows for an estimate of their clinical efficacy.

VITALITY AND PRESERVATION

Like all cells, stem cells require an adequate environment to survive. Outside the body, they die easily. Crowding, pressure, needle gauge, freezing, thawing, and chemical influences (like lidocaine, for instance) are just a few things that are potentially dangerous to stem cells.

Stem cells are at their best when freshly processed. Ideally, they should be used even before the sample is frozen, which requires proximity between the lab and the treatment center.[75] [76] [77]

Although adult stem cell use is prevalent clinically, it represents older technology. However, autologous adult stem cells offer some advantages. There is no need for preservatives; the cells are harvested and promptly administered. Second, the risk of rejection is very low unless mutation or contamination occurs between the harvest and graft. However, this treatment is more expensive than PRP because of the collection process. Up to 40% of bone marrow-derived stem cells are hematopoietic and, therefore, likely of suboptimal efficacy in repairing tissues such as muscles, tendons, and ligaments.

Imperfect harvesting and preservation, including storage at too high a temperature, may be detrimental to stem cell survival. Liquid nitrogen is the standard medium used for cryopreservation, but short-term shipments are made using dry ice.

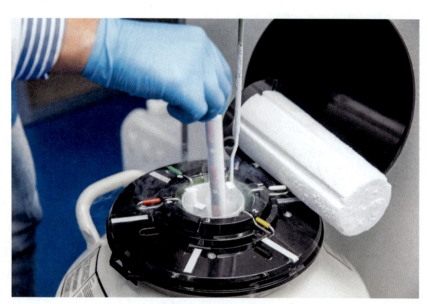

Liquid nitrogen cryotank used to store stem cells

Dimethyl sulfoxide (DMSO), a common preservative, is considered safe by the FDA but is known to be associated with liver and kidney damage. Many laboratories disclose that minimal concentrations of this chemical do not harm stem cells and other companies do not use it because DMSO is cytotoxic in higher concentrations.[78] Though DMSO holds cells stable against cryopreservation (freezing), it may damage preserved cells over the long term.

Nevertheless, per Holm F. et al., contemporary cell freezing techniques offer very good cellular survival without many harmful effects upon subsequent proliferation, "as serum and xeno-free chemically-defined freezing procedures provide over 90% cell viability upon thawing."[79]

Glycerol is another accepted preservative. The major benefit of glycerol as a preservative is the increase in stability and survivability of the stem cells and a reduction of possible systemic reaction compared to DMSO products. This allows for the plausibility of a higher stem cell dose with a lower risk of adverse effects. Glycerol makes the stem cell sample more viscous, sometimes presenting a technical problem when injecting the cells.

Graft-versus-host disease

Graft-versus-host disease is probably the biggest concern for any practitioner who deals with foreign tissue transplants into the human body. Your body can reject even your own autologous stem cells if they develop DNA mutations or if your body has been influenced by toxins, radiation, or nutritional stress. Umbilical cord stem cells, unlike adult stem cells, are immune naive. Lacking immune expression, they are less likely to provoke a response by the recipient's immune system (see "Autologous and allogeneic stem cells" on page 15). In fact, umbilical cord stem cells minimize the active rejection process by repairing inflammation and optimizing the immune system. With time, this property may find an application in post-transplant treatment to improve tissue regeneration and reduce reliance on immunosuppressants when recovering from organ transplants.[80][81][82] Much needs to be done to research and prove the safety of this concept.

Opening the blood-brain barrier

Our brain is protected from chemicals and pathogens penetrating freely into it. This highly sophisticated mechanism exists to shield the central nervous system from potentially toxic substances and infectious agents that can cause injury to the delicate neurons and glia. Made mainly of specialized endothelial cells that line the inner part of the brain's blood vessels, the blood-brain barrier is, in essence, a semi-permeable membrane that regulates the passive and active passage of substances into the brain.

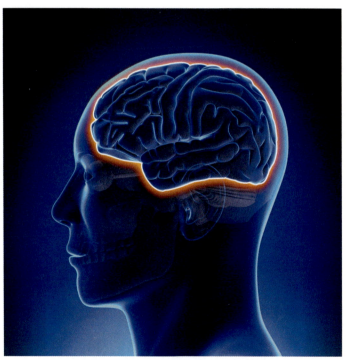

An illustration of the blood-brain barrier

This protective barrier does not appear to allow grafted stem cells to be delivered into the brain when they are infused or injected outside of the central nervous system (outside of the ventricles, the intrathecal space, or brain matter itself) for a variety of possible reasons. As mentioned elsewhere in this book, stem cell secretions are more likely to travel through the blood-brain barrier. Stem cells are potent in their ability to repair the nervous system. Their delivery inside the brain may be desirable in many conditions such as dementia, head trauma, encephalitis, and stroke.

There are indirect ways of bringing stem cells inside the brain by switching off the blood-brain barrier, making it porous. The diuretic mannitol, normally indicated for the treatment of increased intracerebral or intraocular pressure, is known to do this.[83]

The combination of stem cell therapy with mannitol infusions brings stem cells inside the brain, but it can also open the brain to toxins and other unwanted chemicals that would otherwise be kept away.[84] There are many ways to decrease the efficacy of the blood-brain barrier; they include reversing the osmotic opening, focused ultrasound + microbubbles, and through electrical stimulation such as non-thermal electroporation, pulsed electromagnetic stimulation, sphenopalatine ganglion stimulation, and electric field application.[85][86][87][88][89][90][91]

All "brain opening" techniques potentially damage the brain and must not be done routinely. The possible harm frequently outweighs the benefits; this technology is mostly used to treat brain cancer when drug delivery to the brain may prevent an otherwise sure death. Impairing the brain barrier in non-lethal conditions may cause more harm than good.

Host DNA replacement by donor DNA

The question of whether the DNA of a transplanted organ changes to that of the recipient has been answered many times over; no, the organ stays genetically the same and is always seen by the patient's immune system as an invader. Immunosuppression becomes necessary when a patient receives a donor's heart, kidney, or lungs. What about the other way around: would the recipient's body be genetically altered after the donor's organ is transplanted? This concern has been expressed since the early days of organ transplant surgery.

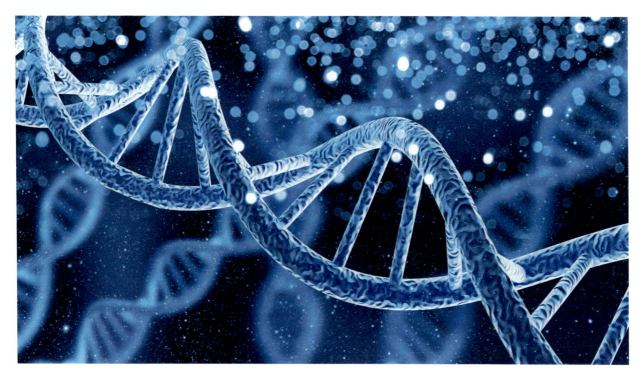

DNA Illustration

A rare case of a transplant patient developing his donor's DNA was reported in Nevada in 2019 when the patient received a bone marrow transplant to treat leukemia. This phenomenon is called "chimera" and is not considered dangerous. Chimeras can also occur naturally; for instance, if a twin dies in the womb and gets "absorbed" by their sibling, or a common phenomenon in pregnant women, if the fetus's cells migrate to the mother's tissue, as reported in Scientific American.[92] A chimera is a single organism made up of cells from two or more "individuals" containing two sets of DNA, with the code to make two separate organisms. In one of the studies, nearly two-thirds of the women were found to have traces of their sons' male Y chromosomes in multiple regions of their brains. "Chimerism" is being actively studied for treating various diseases, most notably Type I diabetes and Alzheimer's disease.

Stem cells from umbilical tissue can potentially do the same thing, and such cases have been described. This phenomenon is called "engraftment" and is not known to present any danger to a stem cell recipient.[93]

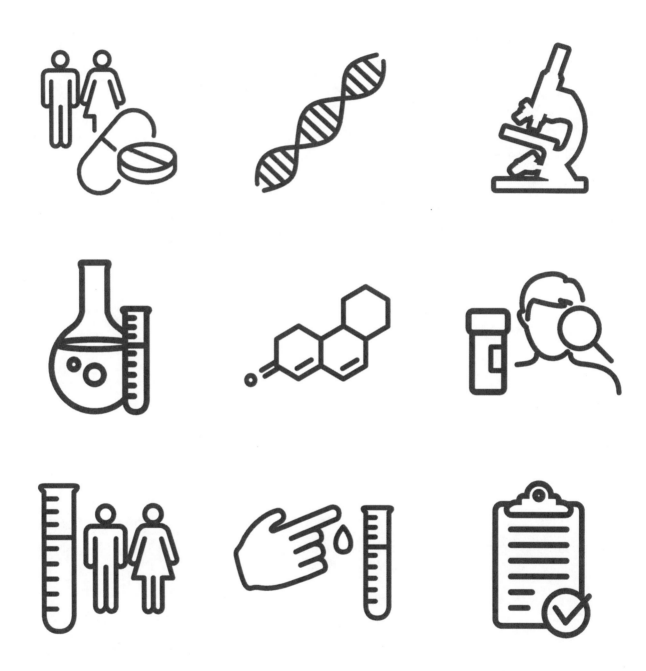

PART THREE:

CLINICAL APPLICATIONS

The clinical applications of stem cells

Although the clinical use of stem cells has been and remains strictly investigational, stem cell treatments were slowly introduced before the latest FDA regulations took effect. The most widespread application was for connective tissue treatments – sports injuries, joint issues, muscle healing, etc. Regenerative medicine has helped establish safety protocols and best practices for delivering stem cell treatment.

Stem cell outcome language is still developing. Do stem cells cure? Do they repair, restore, recover, or improve? All those words may be used, and all the clinical outcomes are possible, including an ambitious definition of "cure." [94] [95] [96]

My clinic has hands-on experience with many conditions, mostly associated with pain. Though the anecdotal experience of clinicians and patients described in this book is relevant and revealing, many more studies must be undertaken to collect and prove the facts before scientifically-based clinical recommendations can be issued. Specific applications of stem cells in clinical practice are not FDA-approved, and they remain experimental and investigational, and many specific methods of administration are also not yet approved. It is prudent to explicitly say that the June 2021 implementation of FDA regulations severely impacted the availability of stem cell and other regenerative treatments in the United States. Budding treatment approaches now need to wait their time to come back into practical medicine. There are exceptions to this rule, and there are always exceptions to the rules!

From now on, I will be explaining what was used in stem cell therapy before these regulations took effect. I hope that future physicians will use this practical knowledge and refine and develop it further. Progress can be slowed but cannot be stopped. Currently stem cell related products are available in many forms, see "Appendix 6: Stem Cell Based Product Classification" on page 90.

Patient experience

Most patients would say their trips to the doctor are boring. Stem cells tend to make appointments more interesting. If the patient receives a stem cell infusion via IV, it starts like any other infusion: a stick in a vein to start an IV. It may not be the most pleasant experience, but it is usually no big deal.

Then comes the exciting part: a frozen vial filled with stem cells. We usually ask the patient to help thaw the vial in the palm of their hand; this can be a good psychological way to "bond" with the stem cells, so to speak. Thawing can also be done in body temperature water or sitting at room temperature until the vial is completely thawed.

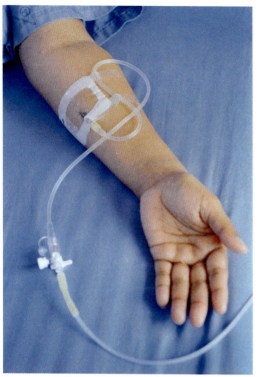

A stem cell intravenous infusion looks and feels no different than any other infusion.

Every vial has an associated tracking number that allows the supplier to trace it back to the source (the donor) should the need for investigation arise. A larger bore needle is used for easier flow and is less traumatic for the stem cells. The cells are introduced into the IV tubing through a slow push from a syringe with normal saline to ensure that almost all cells make it to the patient. Some clinics infuse vitamins and nutrients alongside stem cells. Myer's cocktail – a recipe that varies but usually consists of magnesium, calcium, and vitamins B and C – is popular but tends to be done for psychological reasons rather than proven efficacy. Due to its acidity, vitamin C may not be ideal for use with stem cells, so I would not recommend infusing them together.

Immediate adverse effects are uncommon and are normally associated with the venipuncture rather than stem cells. Some patients experience heaviness in their legs or whole bodies, which is difficult to explain but disappears quickly. A flu-like sensation lasting for a few days has been reported at times.

> **Multiple organ improvement:**
>
> Mrs. E suffered from many chronic conditions, including multiple sclerosis (MS), hypotonic bowel, kidney failure, COPD, fibromyalgia, degenerative arthritis, degenerative disc disease, sacroiliitis (SIJ), and spinal facet disease. She has a complicated medical history that includes two heart attacks and spinal surgery. She was significantly impaired by her combination of diseases but was fortunate to be able to afford repeated stem cell treatments.
>
> After a number of local and systemic (IV) stem cell administrations, her bowel started to work normally; lung and kidney function improved with tests showing diminished pathology; EKG stopped showing post-MI scars on her heart; facets, SIJs and discs became painless; and her knees improved and no longer required replacement as recommended by surgeons before stem cell treatment. Her body pain also disappeared; she is now off the opioids she had been taking for 25 years. Mrs. E's physical health is remarkably better for the past several years. She is not cured, but recurrent stem cell treatment has provided her otherwise unachievable stability.

A specific and frequent reaction was observed in most COVID-immunized patients in our clinic. Stem cell infusions in such individuals produced a reaction that closely mimicked the side effects of an mRNA COVID booster, specifically with a spike of fever, muscle aches, headache, and weakness. This reaction may last anywhere from a few minutes to several hours. It could signify that stem cells produce a similar initial mechanism of immune activation compared to a vaccine—the closer IV stem cell infusion to the time of immunization, the stronger the mentioned adverse effects.

Stem cell injections in joints, muscles, and other body areas are no different from medication injections in those same areas. Stem cells cause initial local (and healthy!) inflammation; temporary swelling can be expected. A day or two of pain increase is also likely. Sometimes the pain may be very pronounced and requires a few doses of oral pain medication, especially when stem cells are introduced into the confined space of a joint. Lidocaine can be used for superficial analgesia, but mixing it with stem cells is contraindicated as lidocaine can kill them. The same goes for steroids. We recommend not using steroids for at least two weeks before and four weeks after stem cell treatment; this applies to both local and IV treatments. However, if the patient's condition does not allow for the discontinuation of steroids, stem cell treatment may still be conducted.

Post-treatment guidelines

In most cases, post-stem cell treatment recommendations are simple: avoid strenuous activity, stay hydrated, and maintain a healthy diet. If problems occur, report them to your doctor as soon as possible.

When stem cells are injected into large joints, additional care is needed. The transplanted stem cells need time before they can tolerate stress.

There is limited published literature about the exact guidelines for physical therapy (PT) after stem cell treatments. The consensus is to avoid high-impact activities for about three months post-injection. The intensity of PT sessions should be reduced by about 25% during the first two weeks and increase slowly over about eight weeks. If the patient lifts weights, decrease the weight by about 25-50%, depending on how heavy the weights were to start with (decrease moderate weights by 25% and heavy weights by 50%) and gradually increase over eight to twelve weeks (see "Appendix 7: Post Treatment Instructions" on page 91).

The question of acupuncture is also open. Acupuncture is unlikely to impede stem cells and may even enhance their function, but electro-acupuncture is controversial. Until more is known, it is probably better to avoid electro-acupuncture, moxibustion, or cupping for at least two to three weeks after stem cell treatment.

Duration of stem cell action

We do not know for sure how long transplanted stem cells live. It depends on the environment they are put in, the diseases the patient has, the kinds of medications the patient is on, and numerous other factors, most of which are unknown at this time.

The duration of stem cell action depends on the cell age at harvest and the transplant niche. Neural tissue, soft tissue, cartilage, and bone have very different local conditions that may significantly limit the possible beneficial effects. Concentrated adult stem cells have therapeutic potential, just not as much as young stem cells (see "Telomeres and aging" on page 22).

What about multiple conditions?

It stands to reason that a patient with 25 diseases would be unlikely to respond to regenerative treatment as well as someone with a single disease (see "What happens to stem cells in the body?" on page 10). Severe diseases will not respond as well as milder conditions. The number of treatments and dosage depends on such factors. The older you are, the more difficult it is to repair tissues. Younger people are expected to improve faster, and the results may last longer. The health of the immune and endocrine systems may aid or impair treatment response.

My patients frequently express surprise that the condition they wanted to treat did not improve as much as some other ailment in their body. We presently cannot direct cells to target a particular problem. Stem cells select their battles for themselves, especially in intravenous administration. A sufficient number of treatments may provide enough cells to attend to most conditions. But stem cells should not be viewed as a cure-all. Repeated treatments are frequently needed, and it is unwise to expect guaranteed recovery.

Stem cells and medications

It is known that lidocaine is toxic to stem cells as it is to many other cells, including cartilage, which complicates tissue injections. Steroids are known to be unsafe in combination with stem cells. Immunosuppressive treatments are not desirable with umbilical cord stem cells but are mandatory with adult allogeneic stem cell transplants.

Cancer treatment medications are designed to kill rapidly-dividing cells and consequently are likely to impair or kill stem cells. Any stem cell treatment on cancer patients, if undertaken at all, should be done between cycles or after the course of chemotherapy or radiation are completed.

Chemicals that change the environment of stem cells, making it too acidic or too basic, would likely interfere with cell vitality and should be avoided.

Intravenous administration

Generalized conditions, especially autoimmune diseases such as rheumatoid arthritis, myasthenia gravis, lupus, Crohn's disease, interstitial cystitis (IC), and others cannot be successfully treated with local injections.[97,98,99,100] The utilization of stem cells, especially blood-derived, also makes sense in uncontrollable infections or hard-to-treat conditions such as Lyme disease. Furthermore, stem cells have been shown to increase egg count and sperm vitality, suggesting their use in infertility problems.[101,102] However, the intravenous route of administration is more controversial and less researched than many other applications. If infused intravenously, stem cells are carried to the lungs, where they settle and multiply for about two weeks. After this time, they leave the lungs and distribute themselves to the areas of need.[103,104,105] This activity has yet to be proven and likely depends on many factors, known and unknown. Other organs such as the gut and spleen may likely filter stem cells and diminish the numbers at the target site. The thymus is also involved in attracting stem cells.

There is a great mystery about the mechanism of stem cell-associated improvement. The treatment does not as much "fix" immune conditions as it modulates them, similar to how a leg prosthesis allows an amputee to walk. Our patients frequently show objective improvement in their autoimmune symptoms without consequent improvement in laboratory markers. The same applies to lung conditions: When a person stops using oxygen, blood oxygen levels normalize while objective lung tests may remain abnormal. The placebo effect can be suspected; however, it cannot explain the sustained improvement in Myasthenia Gravis or increased blood oxygen.

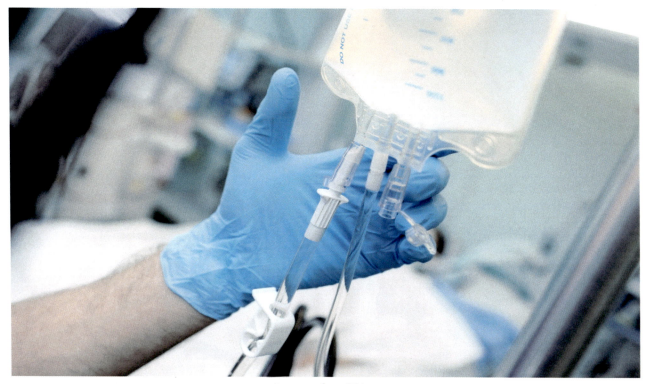

Image of an IV bag

Prophylactic stem cell use, especially in IV formulation, is controversial. It may aid in longevity and illness prevention, though this is highly speculative.

Extracellular products containing no cells but exosomes and exosomal contents are also produced and available. Their potency and usefulness are actively investigated and hold a promise of clinical benefit.

Epidural injections

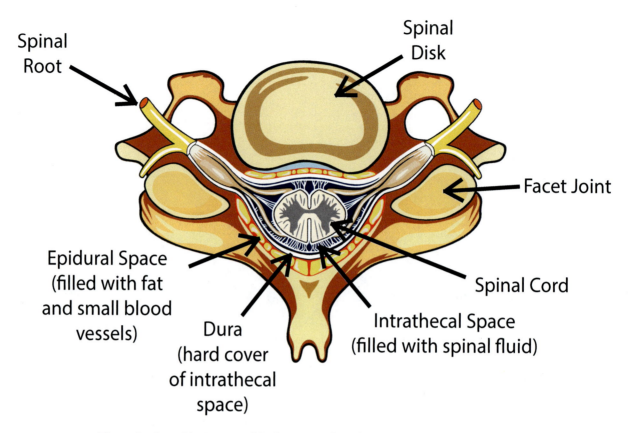

The spinal cord is protected by bones and cushioned by cerebrospinal fluid.

Epidural injections may be considered for spinal root impingement, sciatica, bulging discs, and disc tear repair to replace epidural steroid injections. This is done in clinical practice but is highly experimental and not yet proven.

> Low back pain improvement:
>
> Mr. G suffered from degenerative disc disease (DDD) in his lumbar spine for most of his life. He had several multilevel lumbar spine fusions, spinal cord electronic stimulators, and high doses of opioid medications for decades. His back pain was still not controlled despite already mentioned treatments and many medication combinations in addition to opioids. It seemed he had no hope. It was difficult to expect much improvement in somebody with extensive physical spinal changes and surgeries.
>
> Nevertheless, he dramatically improved after epidural stem cell infusions combined with injections around his discs and implanted instrumentation. Mr. G was weaned off about all of his medications, including complete discontinuation of opioids. It has been several years for him to have as "normal" life as he could have.

INTRATHECAL STEM CELLS

Intrathecal stem cell introduction may be of value due to a theoretically higher penetration into the brain. The cerebrospinal fluid does not float like a river, carrying cells inside the brain. Rather it oscillates up and down. But due to a high concentration in the confined space, intrathecal stem cell introduction has the potential to help with central nervous system diseases such as Parkinson's, Alzheimer's, ALS, Multiple Sclerosis, traumatic brain injury, spinal cord injury, and transverse myelitis.[106][107] As with all stem cell treatments, this remains experimental and potentially riskier that other modes of transplantation.

INTRAARTICULAR ADMINISTRATION

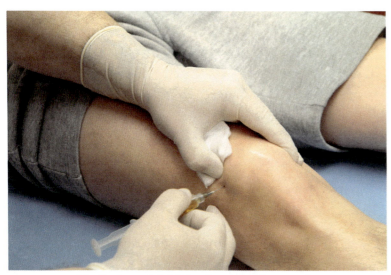

Ideally, knee joint injections are done under fluoroscopic (X-ray) guidance.

The oldest method of stem cell administration is intraarticular (IA/ inside the joint). Like PRP, stem cells treat degenerative joint disease, labrum tears, spine facets, and sacroiliac joints. Clinically, stem cells may be injected directly into the area of trouble with the hope of repair.[108] [109] Some insurance plans (mostly self-insured employer plans) have started to allow coverage of stem cell treatments, especially in the lower extremities and knees.

There is conflicting evidence about what happens to stem cells upon intraarticular injection regarding survivability or destination. There is also conflicting evidence about whether stem cells have a regenerative effect on cartilage. A few studies suggest that there may be some effect. One meta-analysis found no difference in MRI or range of motion in stem cell-injected osteoarthritic knees. At the same time, it did find suppression in pain, suggestive of the anti-inflammatory action of stem cell-secreted molecules.[110]

Just like the patients who, despite abnormal labs, reported improved function of the lungs or immune system, patients who receive intraarticular stem cell treatment frequently report sustained joint pain improvement despite imaging that may still show insufficient cartilage in the joint. We regularly see patients who avoid scheduled joint replacement and show good mobility while their X-rays and MRIs remain suboptimal. Presently we can only speculate how that is possible. We have found that no fluid should be removed or drained from a joint after stem cell injection(s) for at least three months, as this can abruptly stop the healing process and cause increased pain and joint deterioration. If the intraarticular fluid is aspirated earlier, it looks turbid and abnormal, making surgeons suspect an infected/septic knee. Joint fluid culture later comes back negative, but by then, antibiotics are prescribed needlessly, and patients are not happy with the doctor "infecting their knee." The key clinical indicators to differentiate a septic knee from a stem cell caused temporary pain increase are the absence of local redness, lack of fever, and no elevation of white blood cell count.

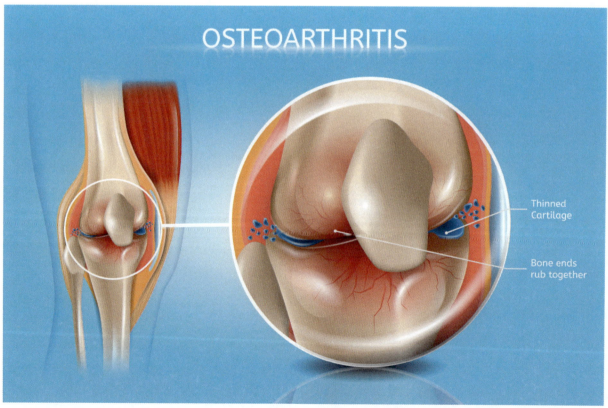

In knees affected by osteoarthritis, the cartilage thins/hardens, fragments break off, bones may develop microfractures, all causing pain. Bringing stem cells into this environment assists in healing and regeneration.

INTRADISCAL INJECTIONS

Intradiscal injections for treating degenerative disc disease, disc tear, bulging, and herniated discs make sense due to the core function of stem cells. Theoretically, mesenchymal cells may be of more value than hematopoietic cells in this application.[111] [112] The efficacy of stem cells for disc injury is not clear with many contradictory studies and little evidence for transplant survival and action of the transplanted cells.

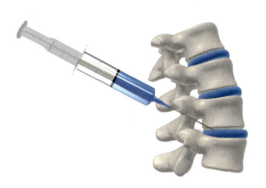

Illustration of an intradiscal injection

The disc is a hypoxic, avascular, and ischemic (poor in oxygen) environment hostile to stem cells. Still, stem cells may assist in regeneration by releasing biologically active factors and improving vascularization and oxygenation of the surrounding tissues. There is a reason to consider injecting only some separated (or synthesized!) growth factors or whole "matrix" into a disk. Several companies are working on bringing these products to the medical market.

Stem cells may also be collected from a healthy nucleus pulposus (the soft inner part of the disc) and injected into a diseased spinal disc. These precursor stem cells are further along the developmental pathway than umbilical cord stem cells. Nucleus pulposus stem cells that were differentiated in a lab setting demonstrated the remarkable but not unpredictable ability to become nerve cells. As such, they have the potential for neural repair in addition to connective tissue repair.[113]

Autoimmune connective tissue disease improvement:

Mr. F was given six months to live. The clinics at Mayo and Stanford had given up on his treatment, both pronouncing that no treatment was available. Mr. F's skin was covered in crust; his immune system malfunctioned severely, making him allergic to about everything; he had neck and shoulder neuropathic pain; severe insomnia and slow deterioration of most of his body. The most sophisticated treatments failed. He came to our clinic with no hope for improvement, rather as due diligence in attending to his condition – which was his natural approach to life.

A combination of local and IV stem cell treatments helped him almost immediately. His neck and shoulder stopped being problematic. His rash dramatically decreased, and his wellbeing improved greatly. Mr. F had several treatments with improvement lasting progressively longer – several weeks, then many weeks, then many months. He is back to an active lifestyle, and his prognosis has changed from death to a full intensity life. However, it will be hard to expect that his symptoms will never return in one way or another.

In August 2019, the FDA granted Fast Track designation for an investigational cell therapy to reduce pain and disability associated with degenerative disc disease. This therapy uses a homologous, allogeneic, injectable cell therapy that utilizes patented progenitor cells, known as discogenic cells. The cells are derived from adult human intervertebral disc tissue and are injected into the target disc. This therapy may have an anti-inflammatory effect and the regenerative capacity to create new intervertebral disc tissue. The FDA is evaluating this product under an investigational new drug allowance and will be regulating it as a drug-biologic through a biologics license application.[114]

Anecdotally, our clinic has observed that placing stem cells around the spinal discs have similar outcomes to injecting the cells inside the discs.

Studying clinical applications is a laborious process and proving the benefits of specific treatments is not easy; this is especially relevant to stem cells.

For instance, one of the latest meta-analyses on intradiscal biologics for low back pain found only low-quality evidence for improvement. A total of 10 observational studies and two randomized clinical trials met the review inclusion criteria in a systematic review performed in 2018 and 2020; they found limited support for intradiscal biologic agent treatment for discogenic low back pain. This review concluded that there might be an application for biologic therapies for discogenic LBP; however, additional, high-quality studies are needed. The explanation that rigorous studies are hard to find is rather simple: the expense and logistics of doing such studies are affordable only to large organizations. Breakthrough research has traditionally been done by small companies or by single individuals, and currently, this path to innovation is suffocated by endless regulation. My readers may understand that an absence of high-quality studies does not mean that the outcomes of smaller studies are invalid. As an oversimplification, you could claim that no rigorous double-blind placebo-controlled studies prove that the sun causes sunburn. Does this dissuade you from thinking that the sun is dangerous for your skin? Blind trust in the scientific process cannot replace common sense.[115]

A recent study published in Scientific Reports compared human umbilical cord-derived mesenchymal stem cells for the treatment of degenerative disk disease and a novel molecular therapeutic "NTG-101" containing a combination of recombinant human Connective Tissue Growth Factor and Transforming Growth Factor beta 1 (TGF-β1). Researchers found that a single injection of NTG-101 into the degenerative disc demonstrated superior benefits compared to stem cell transplantation. Further development of the knowledge of the specific factors involved in an intervertebral disk formation was disclosed in a 2022 review paper, pointing out that "the cellular originators of the intervertebral disc holds vital instructional clues to establish, maintain and possibly regenerate the intervertebral disk." Such incredible advances in the science of regenerative medicine bring us closer to designing medications based on the knowledge of the specific growth factors. Changing to poetic language, I can say that stem cells are the birds, and we, envying them, may one day build an airplane.[116][117]

Intramuscular injections

The intramuscular introduction of stem cells is less controversial than other methods, though still experimental. This treatment has been reported for many high-profile athletes. Autologous stem cells and PRP are also described as beneficial in this application. Nevertheless, the younger the stem cells, the better the potential outcome, so umbilical cord allogeneic cells may still be the choice over autologous adult cells.[118][119][120]

When injected into a large muscle, stem cells can travel some distance around the body. Although transplanted cells may migrate elsewhere, most will concentrate at the injection site to heal the injury. Umbilical cord and placenta-derived acellular factors are currently available for clinical use, including exosomal and matrix products.

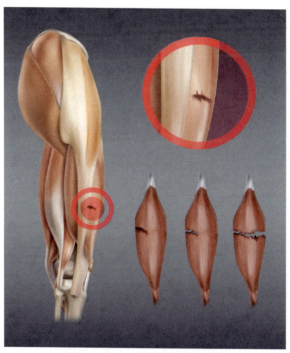

Ruptured muscles heal slowly. Stem cells may help the process.

Intraligament injections

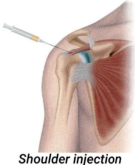
Shoulder injection

Intraligament injections may be considered for Achilles tendon repair, treatment of plantar fasciitis, and knee ligament restoration. Mesenchymal cells may be the right choice in this application.[121][122][123] Acellular stem cell products are destined to be used for this indication.

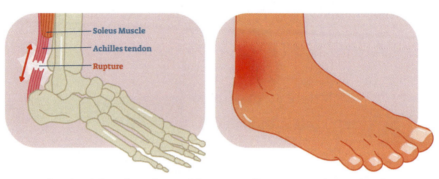

Injecting injured tendons with stem cells may accelerate healing. PRP is also effective for this treatment.

Intraosseous injections

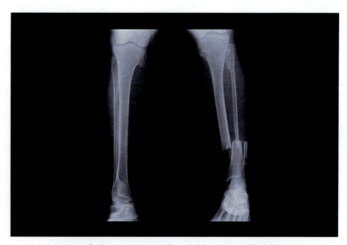
Proof that stem cells aid in bone healing would revolutionize trauma treatment.

Intraosseous (inside the bone) injections for the treatment of bone fractures and non-junction situations (when bones do not come together at the fracture site) are being explored. A new study into parathyroid hormone aiding IV stem cells' ability to home to bone tissue was successful for osteoporosis treatment. Fractures may heal faster; traumas and sports injuries may be amenable to stem cell treatment.[124][125][126] PRP is also actively used for this indication.

Intracardiac injections

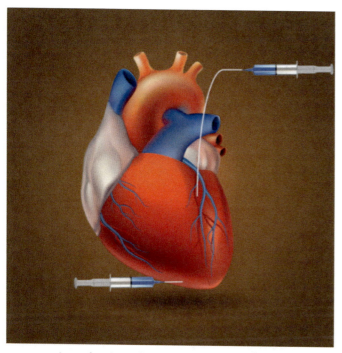
Introduction of stem cells into the heart

Thanks to stem cell migration and homing inside the cardiac wall, cardiac repair after myocardial infarction may be achieved by intracardiac stem cell administration, cardiac artery stem cell infusion, or an IV treatment (it seems all three produce similar results). Much research is going on in this area, but we still do not know enough to be certain of the outcomes of such treatments.[127][128][129][130]

In June 2019, the FDA granted Orphan Drug designation to a cell therapy that delivers allogeneic mesenchymal precursor cells in a single intramyocardial injection. One day this may become a therapy to prevent post-implantation mucosal bleeding in end-stage chronic heart failure patients. This treatment is also investigated in a clinical trial involving moderate to advanced heart failure.[131]

Intraorgan injections

Similar in principle to intracardiac injection, other intraorgan stem cell administration is probably the least researched method, but will likely be of great service to future surgeons once the mechanism and efficacy of such treatments are established. It is not hard to see a future where stem cells are introduced into the pancreas to battle diabetes, or the liver, kidney, or other organs to treat diseases directly.

Brain and intraspinal treatments

Some extracellular components may travel around the body during stem cell migration and cross the blood-brain barrier, but more research must be done to claim this with certainty. We know that stem cells are too big to penetrate the brain when transplanted peripherally, and the best way for stem cells to get inside the central nervous system is through direct introduction. As reported at the American Academy of Neurology 2021 Annual Meeting, stem cell treatment affects outcomes in moderately to severely disabled patients with traumatic brain injury (TBI).[132] No safety concerns related to the stem cells were seen. This report is especially significant because no effective treatments of TBI otherwise exist presently. Patients who received stem cells did statistically significantly better than those who did not. The study's authors suggested that there may be potential for this approach with brain hemorrhage, Parkinson's disease (PD), multiple sclerosis, and other brain-related disorders.

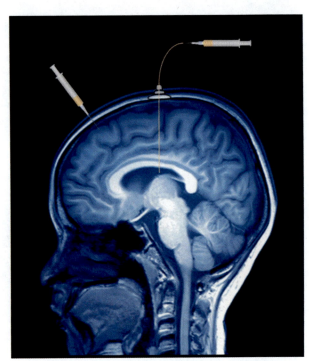

Infusion of stem cells inside ventricles or inside brain matter

Today, brain matter or intraventricular stem cell placement is far from routine clinical practice. One day, stem cells may find their place in neurosurgery, and the same applies to stem cell injections inside the spinal cord to treat severe cord injuries.[133] [134]

At least four cases of spinal tumors have been reported following experimental nasal stem cell transplants for paralysis. The risk of tumorigenesis increases when using an olfactory mucosal autograft, perhaps because the adult autologous cells contain more precursor than progenitor cells; this underlines the cancer risk of adult autologous cells.[135] Your own stem cells might not be as safe as you think.

The biggest problem with stem cells is that they are fragile and may not survive implantation. Emerging technology suggests ways to provide a biologically similar physical and chemical environment to support cells post-administration. According to researchers, bio-inspired hydrogels can be customized to transplant stem cells into most tissue types with a slight modification to the amino acids that make up the target tissue. This technology uses the native proteins present within the implant area and incorporates the most biologically relevant and cell instructive amino acids to form a specialized cell transplantation vehicle.

It is claimed that this hydrogel protects cells during administration and provides an environment after injection that greatly increases their vitality.

> **Post-stroke improvement**
>
> Mrs. H was brought to our clinic by her daughter three years after suffering a left-side stroke. She could not speak coherently (she had fluent aphasia) and could not stand on her own. Her arm had minimal movement, and she could not take care of herself in any meaningful way. The family was interested in possible treatment for the consequences of her stroke.
>
> We cautioned her that it was unlikely that stem cells would offer much, if any, benefit since such a long time had passed after the stroke. Still, Mrs. H's daughter wanted to try as no other reasonable treatments could be offered by modern medicine. Mrs. H received several intrathecal stem cell administrations, which resulted in the family reporting that Mrs. H could stand on her own in the shower. She could move her hand, was more alert, and mentally sharper.

The study authors report that hydrogel tested on mouse brain cells demonstrated that stem cells could be shielded from inflammation and begin to integrate with neural circuitry. By self-assembling into a three-dimensional web that mimics the brain tissue's natural environment, the hydrogel appears to give the transplanted cells a much greater chance of survival.[136]

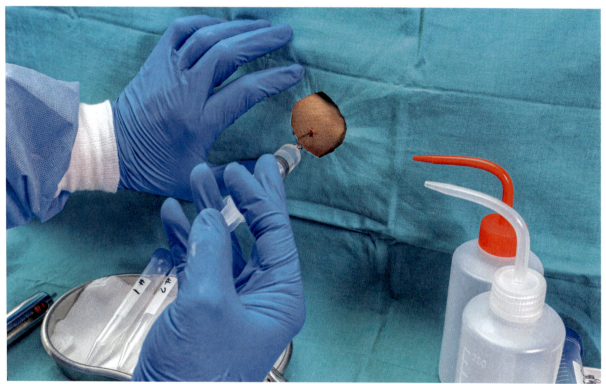

Spine procedure image

Intraocular and eye surface treatment

Intraocular (inside the eye) injections may be disastrous and are not ready for human clinical use. A clinic in Florida was closed by the FDA in 2018 after blinding several patients.[137] However, eye surface treatment is performed successfully by experienced ophthalmologists.[138 139 140] The NIH sponsors ongoing studies of the appropriate use of stem cells in eye diseases.

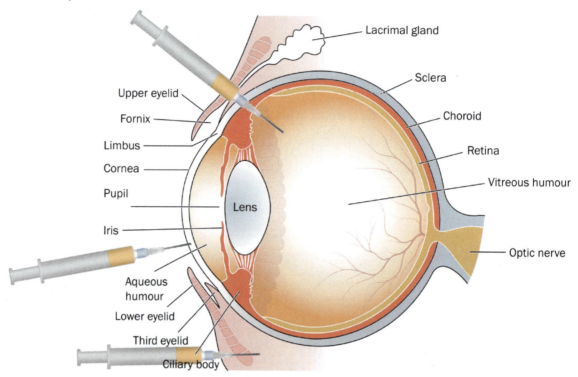

Stem cells may one day be placed in various eye compartments. Much more research has to be done before clinical use is approved.

Intranasal treatment

Allergic rhinitis, sinusitis, trophic mucous ulcers, and other changes may be treated with stem cell products. Spraying live stem cells in the nose does not make much sense because they would quickly die, but acellular preparations such as exosomes and cytokines may be potentially effective thanks to their anti-inflammatory and immune normalizing effects. There is no way to keep stem cells alive in a spray bottle. On the contrary, acellular products require only refrigeration or freezing for longer storage. Continued application of growth factors to the nasal mucus membrane may cause overgrowth; therefore, only short courses, albeit repeated, are recommended.

STEM CELLS AND CANCER

Treating cancer with stem cells is controversial. Although stem cells have been shown to treat multiple types of cancer, there is a danger of giving patients false hope. Costly experimental treatments for life-threatening diseases requires clear and informed patient consent.[141][142][143]

Stem cells may develop into cancerous tumors due to aberrant differentiation. Embryonic stem cells, which have been shown to turn into cancer cells, are considered especially risky from the standpoint of cancer treatment. As mentioned above, there are also reports of adult stem cell involvement in tumorigenesis.[144][145][146] From what is known today, the cancer risk appears lowest with umbilical cord blood and Wharton's jelly stem cells, which so far have not been observed to develop into cancer (see "Amniotic and umbilical stem cell products" on page 20).

Finally, because exosomes are a subset of all of the biologic material found in the umbilical cord, there is also a risk of tumorigenesis caused by the activating factors included within exosomes (see "Exosomes" on page 27).[147][148] The risk heavily depends on the original concentration and activity of the exosomes that are introduced into the patient. This brings an important cautionary note: Too much stem cell treatment may be harmful. You can have "too much of a good thing." Since it is not presently known what is "too much" in relation to stem cells, caution against over-treatment should be the rule for both clinicians and patients. Acellular products derived from placenta and amniotic fluid are safest from a cancer risk standpoint, though they are not normally delivered systemically.

CAN STEM CELLS BE USED TO TREAT PAIN?

There are several ways that stem cells and stem cell products can help with pain. One is immediate, by blocking the initiation of the pain cascade and decreasing inflammation.[149][150] From clinical experience, pain also improves in a delayed fashion and is associated with tissue repair and oxygenation, metabolism improvement, and boosting of the immune system.[151][152][153]

Dental applications

Dental applications of stem cells are expanding, even to the point of growing new teeth. Local dental stem cell injections are logical in both tissue restoration and infection management.[154][155][156][157][158] Acellular products such as placenta-based tissue allografts are ripe to be used in dental transplantations. Synthetic growth factors are also part of the future of dentistry.

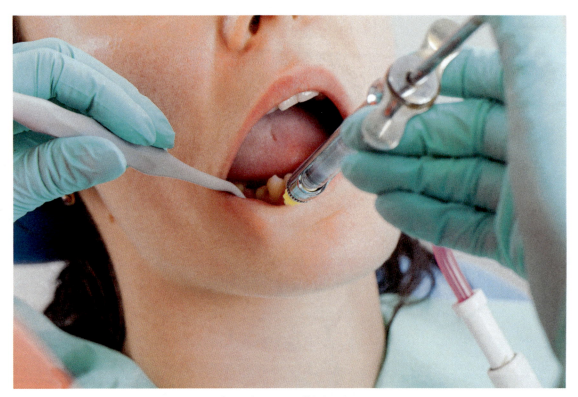

Dental stem cell injection

Cosmetic treatment

The cosmetic use of stem cells is intriguing. One day, there may be a place in medicine to grow and rejuvenate hair, skin, and fat pads.

A large enough needle bore must be used, but scarring from large needle punctures, especially in the face, is of concern. Local anesthetics interfere with stem cell vitality, complicating live stem cell injections in cosmetics. The extracellular component (matrix/exosomes) does not require large-bore needles and may be administered with fine needles.

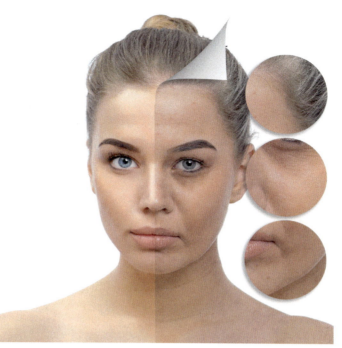

Skin, hair, and fat pad rejuvenation has been reported after stem cell treatments.

The topical use of stem cells for cosmetic purposes is fiction, as live stem cells cannot survive in a cream or an ointment. At the same time, the extracellular component or "serum," to borrow the term used in the cosmetic industry, may be of value if mixed with a chemical vehicle to take growth factors through the skin.[159][160][161]

The most intriguing cosmetic possibility may be through intravenous infusion of stem cells. It is fanciful to contemplate that as stem cells continue to multiply and revitalize within the host – as new tissues replace older ones – stem cell treatments, in a way, make the recipient younger. I am not aware of any human studies looking at this possibility to date. It is unlikely that stem cells can reverse aging. Still, it is probable that the prophylactic use of umbilical cord stem cells, if started early enough, may slow aging and eventually make people appear younger than their calendar age. This has been shown to work in rats.[162] With so many unknowns concerning possible future complications of stem cell treatment, using umbilical stem cells prophylactically is a difficult choice.

Hair color

We have long known that some people's hair rapidly turns gray after they experience extreme stress. Researchers from the Universities of Sao Paulo and Harvard published in the journal Nature that these effects were linked to melanocyte stem cells, which produce melanin and are responsible for hair and skin color.

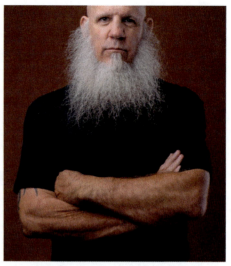

Maybe we can conquer grey.

In experiments on mice, stem cells that control skin and hair color became damaged after intense stress, and the process sped up the depletion of stem cells that produces melanin in hair follicles. Of course, mice are not men, so it is not clear if this finding can be clinically applied to humans, but the fact that stem cells are involved even in hair color is powerful. [163]

Can stem cells prolong life?

A recent study published in the journal *Nature* showed that the aging process might be reversed when stem cells are introduced into a rat's brain, and the cells are then fooled into perceiving that their surroundings are soft and young.[164] The fact that it is possible in rats does not mean that this would directly translate to humans, but the promise is there. We know that stem cells are involved in slowing aging in many different ways.[165]

Other animal studies demonstrate a significant increase in longevity coupled with better health in the experimental subjects. If this effect can be replicated in humans, we may have a better future that requires fewer doctors and hospitals.[166] [167] This is a far-reaching statement but isn't it the ultimate dream?

Growing organs

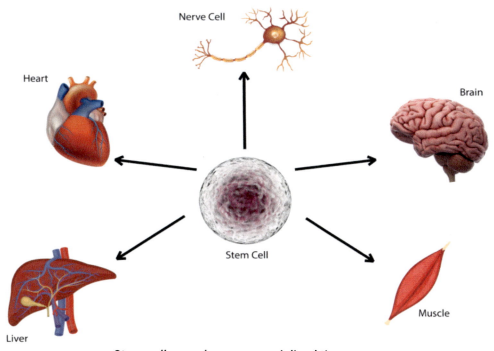

Stem cells may become specialized tissue, opening the door to rebuilding or even replacing damaged organs.

Growing missing organs without stem cell manipulation (presently illegal clinically in the United States) seems impossible, so current clinical stem cell use is confined to repairing preexisting damaged structures. However, with appropriate scientific development, growing healthy organs is possible and will happen in the future.

Scar formation

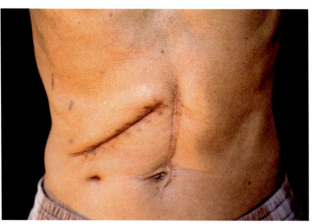

Treating and preventing skin and internal scar formation would help many patients.

Could stem cells be used to treat keloid scars or to prevent post-surgical scarring? [168][169][170][171] Amniotic membrane seeded with stem cells can be used to treat wounds and tissue defects. For example, a successful spina bifida tissue defect repair has been performed,[172] complete with newly- formed sweat glands, seborrheic glands, and hair follicles. The same kind of tissue repair has been seen in animal studies (earhole closure in mice).[173] Stem cells and other stem cell-derived products could also be used to prevent painful adhesions commonly formed after intra-abdominal surgeries.

Mental illness

As we know, multiple mental conditions are based on the inflammatory process. Psychosis, depression, autism, Alzheimer's dementia, traumatic brain injury, and many other diseases are inflammatory in nature. Theoretically, they can be treated with stem cells if it can be conclusively shown that stem cells regulate inflammation. However, this remains speculative at present.[174][175][176][177][178] The use of stem cells has also been reported to treat alcohol and stimulant addiction. Still, the clinical results are far from certain.[179][180] I published an article reviewing stem cell applications in psychiatry if you are interested in learning more.[181]

Stem cells and COVID

Coronaviruses (CoV) are a large family of viruses that cause illness ranging from the common cold to more severe diseases such as Middle East respiratory syndrome (MERS-CoV) and severe acute respiratory syndrome (SARS-CoV). A novel coronavirus (nCoV) is a new strain that has not been previously identified in humans. The current coronavirus disease (COVID-19) pandemic has devastated the world as we know it. In early May 2022, the WHO said that Covid had caused the deaths of more than 15 million people worldwide.

Stem cells seem to be one of the promising treatments actively investigated for use against COVID infection. This approach makes sense because of the core function of stem cells.

COVID-19 comes with a host of symptoms, and they can vary dramatically from patient to patient depending on age, preexisting health factors, and in some cases, for no discernible reason. However, in severe and critical cases, most patients experience what is called a "cytokine storm."

A "cytokine storm" has no firm definition. Instead, it is a general term applied to a situation where the body's immune system improperly releases unregulated cytokines in response to a threat. This condition also goes by several other names, including cytokine release syndrome, hemophagocytic lymphohistiocytosis, and macrophage activation syndrome. Cytokines play an important role in normal immune responses, but having a large amount of them in the body all at once can be harmful.[182]

Stem cells have proven anti-inflammatory capabilities, making them well-suited for treating cytokine storms stemming from COVID-19 and other conditions related to the disease.

As mentioned in *The New York Times*, "Certain kinds of stem cells can secrete anti-inflammatory molecules. Over the years, researchers have tried to use them as a treatment for cytokine storms, and now dozens of clinical trials are underway to see if they can help patients with COVID-19."[183]

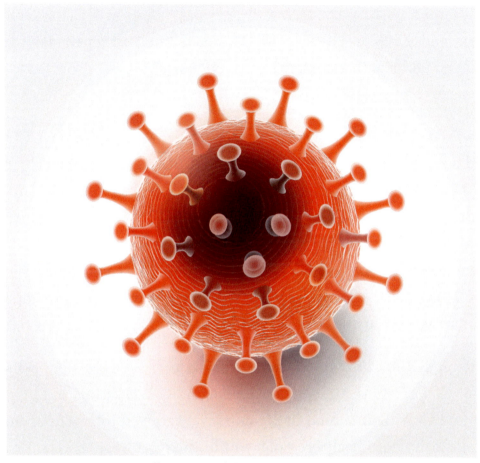

Illustration of the COVID-19 virus

At this time, more than 75 clinical trials are running that involve stem cells to treat COVID-19 symptoms. The sheer number of stem cell-focused trials is a testament to the immense potential offered by mesenchymal stem cells. However, the NYT cautions patients to temper their expectations, saying, "stem cell treatments haven't worked well in the past, and it's not clear yet if they'll work against the coronavirus."

With that being said, stem cell therapy is still very promising. As explained by the authors of the study, *The pathogenesis and treatment of the Cytokine Storm in COVID-19*, published in April 2020, "As an important member of the stem cell family, mesenchymal stem cells (MSC) have the potential of self-renewal and multidirectional differentiation as well as strong anti-inflammatory and immune regulatory functions. MSC can inhibit the abnormal activation of T lymphocytes and macrophages, and induct their differentiation into regulatory T cell subsets and anti-inflammatory macrophages, respectively. It can also inhibit the secretion of pro-inflammatory cytokines, such as IL-1, TNF-α, IL-6, IL-12, and IFN-γ, thereby reducing the occurrence of cytokine storms. At the same time, MSC can secrete IL-10, hepatocyte growth factor, keratinocyte growth factor, and VEGF to alleviate ARDS, regenerate and repair damaged lung tissues, and resist fibrosis. Therefore, many functions of MSC are expected to make it an effective method for the treatment of COVID-19."[184]

Pneumonia and acute respiratory distress syndrome (ARDS) are common in COVID-19 patients, and both conditions reportedly respond to stem cell treatment.[185][186] It has been established that breathing problems respond to stem cell treatment. According to a study titled *Mesenchymal Stem Cell Therapy for COVID-19: Present or Future*, the authors found, "After the intravenous transplantation of MSCs, a significant population of cells accumulates in the lung, which they alongside immunomodulatory effect could protect alveolar epithelial cells, reclaim the pulmonary microenvironment, prevent pulmonary fibrosis, and cure lung dysfunction."[187]

The immune regulation, lung repair and antiviral properties of stem cells are all promising for COVID-19 treatment. As an anecdotal observation, in our practice, we have seen no COVID infection in patients who received intravenous umbilical cord stem cells for various health reasons within the three years before the current pandemic. This could suggest a prophylactic potency of stem cells. Of course, this cannot be scientifically claimed presently and should be thoroughly researched. In December 2021, we had one reported case in this group during the more infective Omicron variant flare-up. The second case was reported in April 2022.

At the end of January 2021, a small California-based company announced positive preliminary results from its study of human allogeneic adipose-derived mesenchymal stem cells for patients suffering from respiratory distress or acute respiratory distress syndrome (ARDS) induced by COVID-19. Intravenous infusion of allogeneic stem cells showed positive results, and the authors reported that infusions were well-tolerated, and no adverse events were observed.[188]

Much more information on the potential use of MSCs for patients with COVID-19 can be found at: https://translational-medicine.biomedcentral.com/articles/10.1186/s12967-020-02380-2

OTHER REGENERATIVE MEDICINE PRODUCTS

The latest regulatory changes limited the production and sales of stem cell-related products. The relatively easy clinical use of stem cells is no longer a reality in the United States. Many companies are currently applying for INDs, and many more applications will be filed in the future.

The fact that an IND is granted does not mean that an authorized product may be used freely; such investigational use comes with many rules, extensive record-keeping, and other burdens. Importantly, studies under INDs are free to the patient, and if anything, patients are sometimes reimbursed for study participation. Understandably, this precludes the commercial use of stem cells. There are likely loopholes around these rules, but this is a legal gray area. Clinics, labs, and clinicians are more likely to get into trouble in gray areas.

Some suppliers of cellular and acellular biologics, however, have continued to make their products available under section 361, allowing easier access to the market. While approved IND applications add legitimacy, vendors are unlikely to sell or market these products outside the IND parameters. Nevertheless, clinical use of any treatment is ultimately the physician's decision with the patient's informed consent.

EMERGING STEM CELL RELATED PRODUCTS

As a result of tightening restrictions on live stem cell preparations, many laboratories are now working on acellular products derived from amniotic fluid and birth waste tissues, including placenta, umbilical cord, and umbilical cord blood.

The extracellular matrix provided by such tissues is easier to control, produce, store, and standardize. They are designed to supplement or replace damaged connective tissue of an adult recipient. The vitality of live cells is not an issue in this process. As a result, such material may be sterilized by gamma radiation while preserving the original characteristics of the donor tissue. I mentioned earlier that FDA regulates these preparations under section 361, 21 CFR 1271.10(a) of the Public Service Act, which guides approval of products that are not drugs, biologics, or medical devices. (www.fda.gov/media/109176/download) This regulation requires products to be minimally manipulated, perform the same function in the recipient as in the donor, be combined only with permitted substances (water, crystalloids, and sterilizing, preserving, or storage agents), and do not have systemic effect nor depend on the metabolic activity of live cells.[189] This is different from complex biological products regulated under section 351, which has to follow the standards of the medication approval process and allows products to be manipulated, may have a systemic effect, and be studied only under government-granted IND application.

Described as "Acellular Placental Extracellular Matrix Allograft" (ECM), such human tissue therapy products contain regenerative factors that may assist in regulating inflammation, tissue formation, and remodeling. As a result, these products locally support the recipients' cells and cellular activity. Like live stem cells, they are collected from full-term elective cesarian section delivery with full donor consent and are screened per FDA guidelines.

Examples of acellular products

Several general product lines are currently enjoying lesser regulation in the US:

- **Lyophilized Amniotic Membrane** may be used as a natural barrier for application on non-healing wounds such as diabetic and venous leg ulcers and pressure wounds. Healing of surgical non-pathologic wounds also may be assisted by applying amniotic membrane. They come in various sizes and are designed to cover damaged skin.[190] Amniotic membrane products are minimally manipulated and processed to preserve the original relevant characteristics. Such products have been used clinically for over 100 years, with more than 100 publications devoted to them over time.

- **Amniotic fluid-derived products** contain billions of exosomes, extracellular vesicles filled with hundreds of cytokines, growth factors, and hyaluronic acid. Free-floating cytokines and growth factors also may be collected from amniotic fluid and used therapeutically.

- **Blood-derived products.** Material for these products is easily harvested using established protocols with high viability. One of the companies, Lucina BioSciences, developed an interesting acellular product that allows binding platelets from PRP. This holds them in place, preventing migrating and diffusing away from a treatment site. Platelets are activated after binding to local body tissue and secrete soluble factors from their intracellular granules.[191][192][193][194] In theory, this improves tissue healing and regeneration by preserving a higher concentration of the active ingredient, platelets, in the target area.[195]

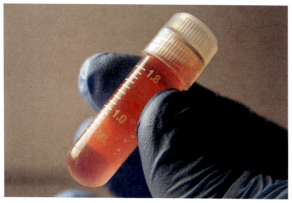
Example of blood-derived product

- **Placenta and umbilical cord-derived products.** The source of tissue for placenta-derived tissue allograft is easy to acquire. It contains many components imperative for developing the foundational extracellular matrix, such as collagen, which forms fibrils that provide structure for soft tissues like ligaments, tendons, and skin. It naturally contains the necessary ingredients for developing an extracellular matrix that helps to assist with the repair, reconstruction, and supplementation of the recipient's tissues. The placental tissue serves as a viable platform for the body's healing components to work together within the matrix to regulate inflammation and initiate cell regrowth within the tissue. A tissue allograft scaffold utilizes a naturally formed mixture of bioactive molecules and precursors found in placental tissue. By administering the tissue allograft into defected body area, a new 3D structure of healthy tissue can be regenerated.[196][197][198] The company, producing placental-derived tissue allograft published a technical statement, outlying contents of the product. It contains a large number of active amniotic membrane composites that may be found in "Appendix 8: Placental-Derived Tissue Components" on page 92.

- **Minimally processed birth waste (MPBW).** This is relatively new, with very few manufacturers. The combination of the various components has demonstrated superior clinical efficacy. The inclusion of the serum and other sources improves post-thaw viability and stability. It is unclear under which regulatory category these products will fall and how difficult it would be to introduce them to the medical market.

There are many INDs granted by the government so far, and they cover a wide array of applications. One of the companies, Organicell Regenerative Medicine, is especially active in the field and has INDs granted for the treatment of SARS due to COVID-19, the use of acellular biologic in prolonged COVID-19, the treatment of chronic obstructive pulmonary disease (COPD), and the treatment of osteoarthritis.

Cord blood vs. tissue allografts

Umbilical cord blood is a tissue product; it contains all the normal elements of blood - red blood cells, white blood cells, platelets, and plasma. If done correctly, it also contains PRP from birth waste. It is rich in blood-forming stem cells, similar to those found in the bone marrow. The FDA classifies it as Human Cell, Tissue and Cellular and Tissue-Based Products regulated under section 351 of the Public Health Service Act (PHS).

On the contrary, the FDA classifies tissue allografts as tissue-based products. Such acellular placenta-derived tissue derivatives are not blood and do not contain live, viable cells or normal blood elements like red and white blood cells, platelets, and plasma. These products are regulated under section 361 of the PHS Act. Tissue allografts are comprised of extracellular matrix (ECM) derived from non-amnion placental tissue. It is intended to serve as a scaffold that provides physical support and tissue cushioning while serving as a conduit that connects and supports cellular activity. Tissue allografts are exempt from the FDA pre-market review, clearance, and approval, making them cheaper to manufacture and more affordable to the labs, physicians, and patients alike. They are still innovative therapies based on medical necessity, though their therapeutic value is likely less than full cellular products. Acellular products are a good practical choice in today's market.

In addition to better affordability, one of the critical advantages of tissue-derived products is that they can be stored at room temperature and have a shelf life of several years.

It is important to remember that, as with the implantation of any human tissue, there is always the possibility of an allergic reaction or transmission of infectious disease, even with the best preventive measures.

Conclusion

A new field of knowledge is always exciting. One feature is common in anything new and unexplored: difference in opinions, which is usually enriching and positive but is sometimes bitter and toxic. Extremists claim that only their opinion matters when, in fact, every approach is useful, depending on the circumstances. Applied to regenerative medicine, this means that PRP, amniotic fluid, amniotic membrane, exosomes, matrix, autologous, and allogeneic stem cells all have practical uses. We should be wary of those who claim that only one product or modality has any value, and, of course, everything has to be appropriately investigated.

So much about the world of stem cell treatment and regenerative medicine remains unknown. We still need to learn who to treat, what kind of stem cell products to use, and what indications stem cells may treat. The timing of stem cell treatment based on the patient's age and disease process remains unclear. The question of treatment boosters is still open. Should we wait until the patient's disease relapses, or should we repeat treatment before their disease worsens? Combination treatment with medications is also unclear. Which medications aid or impair the efficacy and safety of stem cells? What about electric, mechanical, or magnetic stimulation of tissues with stem cells? Do vitamins and nutrients affect stem cell function? If so, how? When are live stem cell treatments preferable, and when are acellular products more beneficial? Years of research are needed to answer these and other questions. Hopefully, more research will help us maximize the safety and efficacy of stem cells in clinical practice.[199,200,201,202]

Innovation in medicine comes from both laboratory and clinical practice. Thousands of stem cell studies are underway around the world, half of them in the United States. Adult stem cells, allogeneic stem cells, Wharton's jelly, and cord blood are being actively studied (see "Appendix 9: Current Stem Cell Studies" on page 93).

In 2020, China issued draft regulations that would permit some hospitals to market therapies developed from the patient's own cells, without approval from the nation's drug regulator. The International Society for Stem Cell Research (ISSCR) sent a statement outlining its concerns to China's National Medical Products Administration in Beijing, urging more research before the wide use of these therapies. This development points to a fragile balance of countervailing forces: innovation and regulation, efficacy and safety, medical and political – in short, risk and reward. As presented earlier, the FDA clamped down on the clinical application of stem cells in the USA outside of INDs, sharply slowing the development of the regenerative medicine field.

There is no easy match for the promise and pitfalls of stem cell research and treatment. The pharmaceutical model, which zeros in on a single molecule for exhaustive testing, does not apply to complex biological products such as stem cells. Governments do not know how to assure safety without suffocating fact-finding in stem cell research. A national registry is needed. Clinical outcomes need to be reported and analyzed. Stem cell laboratories need to be systematically reviewed and compared transparently and understandably. Patients need to be able to find appropriate treatment. Doctors, regulators, and the public need education. This requires deep reservoirs of scientific brainpower, organizational genius, institutional and political goodwill, and sufficient funding.

And yet the endeavor is worth the expense. We are constantly enriched by new knowledge, and the clinical use of stem cells opened new horizons before the supply was cut off in the US. Stem cell treatment was reserved for otherwise untreatable conditions; our knowledge base and experience expanded. We will likely witness a healthcare revolution when the regulatory environment improves.

Stem cell science develops quickly, and what seems to be true today may not be true tomorrow. This book is a good example: the second edition, just one year after the first publish, contained many new chapters, additions, corrections, and clarifications. This third edition follows changes witnessed since 2020. This is the nature of science; learning is a lifelong project. This edition reflects what is known at the time of writing. I hope it will be a stepping stone for those who continue to be interested in stem cells and the field of regenerative biologics.

PART FOUR:

END MATTER

Appendix 1: Selected Stem Cell Glossary

Term	Definition
allogeneic stem cells	stem cells from a donor other than the recipient
allograft	donor tissue collected from the same species
amniotic fluid	the liquid that cushions a growing fetus; it lacks live stem cells but is rich with cytokines and growth factors produced by stem cells
amniotic membrane	the lining of the embryonic sack; it is covered with stem cells and may be used topically as a healing barrier treatment for burns, wounds, etc.
animal stem cells	any animal tissue-derived stem cells
autologous stem cells	the patient's own stem cells used on him or herself
embryonic stem cells	stem cells derived from aborted embryos; the source of serious moral, ethical, and religious concerns; today no embryonic stem cells are permitted for clinical use in the United States
exosomes	cellular sub-compartments of living cells; packaged with payloads of growth factors, cytokines, & other factors designed to secrete from the cells and released into the extracellular environment
hematopoietic stem cells	stem cells that are present primarily in blood and bone marrow; they differentiate into white and red blood cells and plasma components which aid the immune system; lymphocytes, monocytes, and macrophages also come out of this cell line, aiding in anti-inflammatory processes in the body
matrix (fibrose)	matrix lacks a precise definition and usually refers to an assembly of mostly fibrose proteins and cytokines from stem cells with no actual live stem cells in the composition
mesenchymal stem cells	these stem cells may come from anywhere in the body, but are especially prevalent in the umbilical cord wall; these stem cells mostly differentiate into connective tissue and are involved in organ repair
precursor stem cells	stem cells than can become a cell or a tissue of a particular type (i.e., ligaments, muscles or cartilage, and not endocrine cells)
progenitor stem cells	stem cells than can become almost any cell or tissue with a preference for certain tissue types (i.e., mostly connective tissue with some blood cells)
PRP	platelet-rich plasma is not stem cells or matrix per se; it is the activated expression of a host of growth factors secreted by platelets that, in turn, act upon the tissue target, such as tendon or ligament
totipotent stem cells	stem cells (only present in blastocyst) that can become any cell or any tissue
umbilical cord blood stem cells	mostly hematopoietic stem cells that are especially suitable for becoming blood cells and immune regulators
umbilical cord stem cells	stem cells collected from the donated birth waste of healthy live newborns; umbilical cord stem cells are undifferentiated and to date have not been associated with oncogenesis, nor do they turn into cancer
umbilical cord wall stem cells	mostly mesenchymal stem cells that are especially suitable for becoming connective tissue

Appendix 2: Notable Dates

1868	German scientist Valentin Häcker coins the term "stammzelle" (German for stem cell)
1908	Russian scientist Alexander Maksimov and others use the term "stem cell" for their work in hematopoiesis
1963	McCulloch and Till (Ontario Cancer Institute Canada) illustrate the presence of stem cells in mouse bone marrow
1968	First bone marrow transplant between siblings with severe comorbid immunodeficiency (SCID)
1974	First report on stem/progenitor cells in human cord blood.
1981	Gail Martin (UCSF) isolates stem cells from a mouse embryo
1988	First successful cord blood transplant to regenerate blood and immune cells in Paris, France on a six-year-old boy suffering from Fanconi's Anemia (from identical twin sister)
1991	Dr. Arnold Caplan coins the term "mesenchymal stem cell."
1992	New York Blood Center establishes the first public CB bank.
1993	First unrelated allogeneic (UCB) transplant performed
1996	First unrelated (allogeneic) cord blood transplant in adults
1998	Netcord group is created in Canada to establish good practices in umbilical cord blood banking, and the first successful transplant is conducted to cure sickle cell anemia
2001	Research shows that cord blood is a suitable alternative to adults requiring a stem cell transplant
2003	Successful stem cell treatment after stroke
2006	Research increases in the use of cord blood to treat autoimmune diseases and brain disorders
2011	Ministers of Health announce Canada's first national, publicly-funded umbilical cord blood bank managed by Canadian Blood Services
2012	Clinical trial for autism treated with self-cord blood stem cells begins in Sutter Neuroscience Institute, Sacramento, California
2012	It is estimated that more than 35,000 cord blood transplants have been performed worldwide
2015	Along with cord blood, Wharton's jelly and the cord lining have been explored as sources for mesenchymal stem cells (MSC) and had been studied in vitro (in a laboratory), in animal models, and early-stage clinical trials for cardiovascular diseases, as well as neurological deficits, liver diseases, immune system diseases, diabetes, lung injury, kidney injury, and leukemia
2017	Over a million stem cell transplants have been recorded worldwide
2020	Investigation of the use of stem cells to treat COVID
2021	FDA implements changes to regenerative medicine regulation

History develops quickly, and we are destined to see many advances and discoveries, clinical applications, and, of course, more specific regulations ahead of us. Health care historians will eventually systematize and streamline major milestones of stem cell history. I challenge them to do this sooner rather than later.

Appendix 3: Amniotic Product Components

Example Components of Amniotic Products

General Cytokines:
    Fetuin-A
    Interleukin 37
    Macrophage Colony
    Serpin A4
    Syndecan - 4

Growth Factor Cytokines:
    Bone Morphogenic Protein - 7
    Complement Component 5a
    Fibroblast Growth Factor
    Platelet-Derived Growth Factor
    Thrombospondin - 2

Scaffolding Cytokines:
    Adhesion G Protein
    Collagen 1,2,3
    Elastin
    Fibronectin
    Hyaluronic Acid

Homeostatic Cytokines:
    Cystatin - B
    Galectin - 9
    Granulysin
    Lipocalin - 2
    Syndecan - 4

Products are processed from donated human tissue from full-term deliveries following FDA guidelines.

Source: Predictive Biotech

Appendix 4A: Growth Regulating Factors

Selected Growth Factors secreted by Stem Cells[203]		
Paracrine factor	**Organ/Disease**	**Function**
Ang1 and Ang2 (angiopoietins)	Heart, wound healing	Angiogenesis
bFGF (basic fibroblast growth factor)	Heart, wound healing, bone, nervous system	Cardio protection, angiogenesis, granulation tissue formation, capillary formation, bone formation and repair, neuroprotection
BMP-4 (bone morphogenic protein)	Bone, nervous system	Determines NSC, NPC, bone formation and repair
BDNF, GDNF	Nervous system	Protects motor neurons, increased D neuron survival
IGF-1	Nervous system, heart	Protects motor neurons, cardio protection, angiogenesis, recruits progenitor cells, activates CSC
IL-7	Bone marrow	Supports hematopoiesis
MMPs (matrix metalloproteinase)	Heart, bone, cancer	Establishes ECF homeostasis, inhibits fibrosis, regulates bone ECM, tumor growth and migration
NGF	Nervous system	Increased D neuron survival, delineates the lineage specification for NSC and NPC
NT-3 (neurotrophin)	Nervous system	Survival and differentiation of existing and new neurons and synapses
TNF-alpha	Heart	Angiogenesis

Appendix 4B: Immune Regulating Factors

Selected Immune Regulating Factors secreted by Stem Cells[203]		
Paracrine factor	**Organ/Disease**	**Function**
HGF	Immune system, heart, wound healing	Inhibits T-cell proliferation, cytokine production and cytotoxicity, recruits progenitor cells, activated cardiac stem cells, granulation tissue, capillaries formation
IDO (indoleanine 2,3 dioxygenase)	Immune system	Inhibits T – and NK cells, cytokine production and cytotoxicity, mediates T-cell apoptosis
IL-1	Immune system, heart	mediates T-cell proliferation, cardio protection, neurogenesis
IL-6	Immune system, bone marrow, cancer	Mediates T- and B-cell proliferation, protects dendrites and neutrophils, role in tumor growth and migration
TGF-beta	Immune system, heart, bone	Inhibits T- and NK-cell proliferation, cytokine production and cytotoxicity, inhibits fibrosis; bone formation and repair

Appendices 4A and 4B refer to the same Endnote.[203]

Appendix 5: Section 351 vs. 361 Flowchart

Section 351 vs. 361 Flowchart

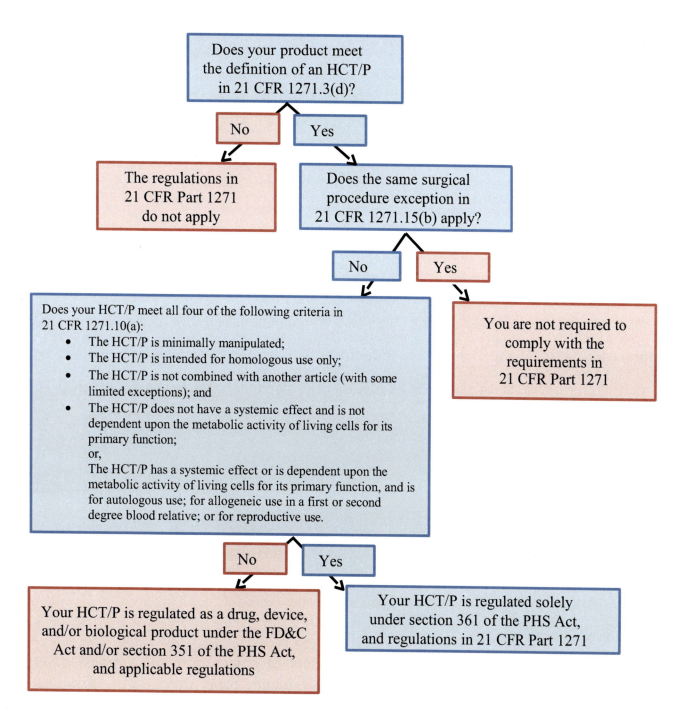

Source: Regulatory Considerations for Human Cells, Tissues, and Cellular and Tissue-Based Products: Minimal Manipulation and Homologous Use, FDA July 2020

Appendix 6: Stem Cell Based Product Classifications

Cellular products

Live stem cells – allows for possible extension in the recipient, cell-to-cell interaction, and continued secretory activity

- *Allogeneic stem cells – from birth waste material*
    - Mesenchymal (mostly cord wall) cells – best for tissue regeneration
    - Hematopoietic (mostly cord blood) cells – best for autoimmune augmentation
    - Mixed mesenchymal and hematopoietic cells – maximize the functions of both types
    - Stem cells sourced from the placenta
- *Allogeneic adult stem cells – from adult donors*
    - May come from bone marrow, adipose tissue, or other adult tissue
- *Autologous stem cells – from the recipient's own tissue*
    - May come from bone marrow, adipose tissue, or other adult tissue
- *Embryonic stem cells – sourced from aborted embryos (not used clinically)*

Other allogeneic (no guaranteed vitality) cellular products from birth waste material

- *Cells from these products act like containers carrying loads of active factors to the recipient*

Stem cells modified and extended outside the body – enhanced for a specialized purpose

Induced pluripotent stem cells (iPSC) – mature cells manipulated to become stem cells

Acellular products

Exosomes

- *Derived from birth waste material – avoiding whole cells reduces cost and tumorigenesis risk and makes transportation and storage easier*
    - A mixture of exosome material
    - Selected exosomes – chosen to produce specific actions
- *Exosomes derived from adult tissue*
    - May be a mixture of exosome material or selected exosomes

Cytokines/Growth Factors

- *Derived from selected birth waste components to standardize and streamline specific desirable actions – lower cost and tumorigenesis risk and easier storage and transportation*
- *Derived from adult tissue*
- *A mix of cytokines/growth factors and fibrous elements (matrix)*
- *Synthetic cytokines/growth factors*

Appendix 7: Post Treatment Instructions

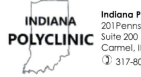

Indiana Polyclinic
201 Pennsylvania Pkwy
Suite 200
Carmel, IN 46280
☏ 317-805-5500

Regenerative Biologics
POST INFUSION/INJECTION INSTRUCTIONS

PATIENT COPY

IV Regenerative Biologics Treatment
Heaviness in the body and flu-like sensations have been reported. This is normal, may last for 1-3 days and no action is needed.

> If the patient experiences fever or other severe unexpected complications, contact your doctor and/or seek emergency (ER) treatment.

Epidural/Intrathecal Regenerative Biologics Administration
Heaviness in the body and flu-like sensations have been reported. This is normal, may last for 1-3 days and no action is needed.

> Fever, paralysis, severe headaches, seizures, and other severe symptoms are not expected - however, if the patient should experience any of these, they should immediately seek emergency (ER) treatment.

Regenerative Biologics Treatment Joint Injections
Heaviness in the body and flu-like sensations have been reported. This is normal, may last for 1-3 days and no action is needed.

Swelling of the injected joint is common and can be severe. As long as there is no redness and fever, even significant swelling is OK. Gentle ice application and elevation of the extremity helps.

Pain in the injected joint is also common and can be severe. Without other symptoms, significant pain does not indicate that something is wrong.

Post procedure, fluid in the joint should not be removed (drained). Doing so can cause the healing process to stop abruptly, making joint disease/pain worse.

> If the patient experiences fever or other severe unexpected complications, contact your doctor and/or seek emergency (ER) treatment.

For mild to moderate pain and swelling patients may use Tylenol alone. For severe pain, patients may need Tylenol 1000mg in combination with ibuprofen 800mg up to three times a day. The more swelling and pain, the more ibuprofen is needed. Sometimes the pain may be severe enough that a few doses of an opioid medication may be needed. Anti-inflammatory medications such as ibuprofen may negatively affect regenerative biologic products shortly after their introduction in the joint and, when possible, should be avoided.

Physical Therapy (PT) and exercise after regenerative biologics joint treatments
Avoid high impact activities for about 3 months post-injection (such as running, etc.) PT sessions are recommended to be reduced in the strenuousness of the session by about 25% during the first 2 weeks and increase slowly over the course of about the next 8 weeks. If you lift weights, reduce the weight by about 25-50% depending on how heavy the weights were to start with (moderate weights - 25% / heavy weights - 50%) and increase over the course of 8 to 12 weeks.

Acupuncture and other alternative treatments after a regenerative biologics treatment
Acupuncture is unlikely to impede and actually may enhance their function. The use of electro-acupuncture after such treatments is controversial. Until more is known, it is probably better to avoid electro-acupuncture, moxibustion, or cupping for at least 2-3 weeks post treatment.

© 2022, Indiana Polyclinic

MR#: 5019

Appendix 8: Placental-Derived Tissue Components

Placental-Derived Tissue Allograft Components

General Amniotic Membrane Composition
Electrolytes
Amino Acids
Cytokines
Hormones
Lipids
Carbohydrates
Urea

Growth Factors in Amniotic Membrane
Platelet Derived Growth Factor (PDGF)
Epidermal Growth Factor (EGF)
Transforming Growth Factors (TGF)
Insulin Like Growth Factor-I, -2 (IGF-I, -2)
Hepatocyte Growth Factor (HGF)
Fibroblast Growth Factor (FGF)

Extracellular Matrix Elements in Amniotic Membrane
Hyaluronic Acid
Tissue Inhibitor of Metalloproteinases (TIMPs)
Fibronectin
PDGFRα
Periostin
Lysozyme
Lactoferrin
Transferrin
Peroxidase
Immunoglobulin G (IgG)
Human Serum Albumin (HSA)

Placental-derived natural tissue allografts are procured through voluntary donation from scheduled Caesarean procedures of healthy full-term births. Maternal donors are screened per FDA and AATB guidelines for a panel of infectious diseases at an FDA registered and CLIA Certified laboratory and against established medical-social risk factors.

Source: Cellulam Core, LLC.

Appendix 9: Current Stem Cell Studies

STUDY SEARCH TERM	STEM CELL STUDIES UNITED STATES	TOTAL
Stem Cells	2906	6182
Mesenchymal stem cells	202	1113
Hematopoietic stem cells	1872	3285
Umbilical cord stem cells	70	330
Umbilical cord blood stem cells	88	114
Exosomes	27	127
Cytokines	443	1416
Growth factors	758	1825

Source: ClinicalTrials.gov (as of May 1, 2022) - includes completed and withdrawn studies

Acknowledgments

My deepest gratitude goes to the patients who underwent stem cell treatments and shared their experience with me. I must thank my friend, publisher, and stickler to English rules Paul Adams, whose contribution is invaluable. Thank you, Dr. Mark Erwin, of Notogen Inc., and the University of Toronto, for providing the insightful critique of a cellular scientist; Drs. Eliott Spenser of Utah Cord Blood Bank and Atta Behfar of the Mayo Clinic, whose knowlege of exosomes shaped my insight; Stu Bowes, who applied a decisive push to dump me into the turbulent waters of stem cells; Dr. Ursula Jacob, my first stem cell teacher; Dr. Scheffer Tseng, whose innovation in stem cell science is impossible to overestimate; Lily Hills who helped me name the first edition; Anthony Gattone for his wisdom on religion; Indiana Polyclinic doctors Rachel Boggus and Brian Paquette who skillfully and successfully do every day what others would dream doing once in a lifetime. The countless animals who give their lives for us to know more about the world have to be profoundly thanked. And I am endlessly thankful to my family and friends to whom this little book is devoted.

ENDNOTES

1. Adapted from Nathan and Ding. Cell, 140:871-882, 2010
2. Zimmerman A, Jyonouchi H, Comi A, et al. Cerebrospinal Fluid and Serum Markers of Inflammation in Autism, Pediatric Neurology, (Sept 2005);33(3):195-201
3. Bergin V, Gibney S, Drexhage H. Autoimmunity, Inflammation, and Psychosis: A Search for Peripheral Markers, Biological Psychiatry (February 2014);75(4):324-331
4. Miller A, Raison C. The role of inflammation in depression: from evolutionary imperative to modern treatment target . Nat Rev Immunol. January 2016; 16(1): 22–34
5. Hwang SH., Kim MH., Yang IH et al., Analysis of cytokines in umbilical cord blood-derived multipotent stem cells. Biotechnology and Bioprocess Bioengineering. 2007,12:32-38
6. E. Soleymaninejadian, K. Pramanik, and E. Samadian, Immunomodulatory properties of mesenchymal stem cells: cytokines and factors. American Journal of Reproductive Immunology. 2012;67(1):1-8
7. Dvorak HF, Tumors: wounds that do not heal. Similarities between tumor stroma generation and wound healing N Engl J Med. 1986 Dec 25; 315(26):1650-9
8. Abbott JD, Huang Y, Liu D, Hickey R, et al. Stromal cell-derived factor-1alpha plays a critical role in stem cell recruitment to the heart after myocardial infarction but is not sufficient to induce homing in the absence of injury. Circulation. 2004 Nov 23; 110(21):3300-5
9. Zhang HT, Fan J, Cai YQ, Zhao SJ, Xue S, Lin JH, Jiang XD, Xu RX. Human Wharton's jelly cells can be induced to differentiate into growth factor-secreting oligodendrocyte progenitor-like cells. Differentiation. 2010;79:15–20
10. Campard D, Lysy PA, Najimi M, Sokal EM. Native umbilical cord matrix stem cells express hepatic markers and differentiate into hepatocyte-like cells. Gastroenterology. 2008;134:833–848
11. Dellavalle A, Maroli G, Covarello D, Azzoni E, Innocenzi A, Perani L, et al. Pericytes resident in postnatal skeletal muscle differentiate into muscle fibres and generate satellite cells. Nat Commun. 2011;2:499
12. Memorial Sloan Kettering Cancer Center. Allogeneic Stem Cell Transplant: A Guide for Patients & Caregivers, 2017
13. Jennifer Choi. Assimetric cell division: its implication for stem cells and cancer. February 24, 2017 Biol 312 @UNBC – Molecular cell physiology
14. Arutyunyan I, Elchaninov A, Makarov A, Fatkhudinov T. Umbilical Cord as Prospective Source for Mesenchymal Stem Cell-Based Therapy. Stem Cells International Volume 2016, Article ID 6901286
15. Andrew S. Rowlands et al. Am J Physiol Cell Physiol 2008;295:C1037-C1044
16. Marie-Luce VIGNAIS. Role of mesenchymal stem/stromal cells (MSCs) in the microenvironment. Model system: interactions between MSCs and cancer cells. Regulation of the energetic metabolism. INSERM U1183 "Cellules Souches, Plasticité Cellulaire, Médecine Régénératrice Et Immunothérapies"
17. https://phys.org/news/2015-04-age-discrimination-cell-division-stem-cells.html#jCp
18. Fong CY, Gauthaman K, Cheyyatraivendran S, Lin HD, Biswas A, Bongso A. Human umbilical cord Wharton's jelly stem cells and its conditioned medium support hematopoietic stem cell expansion ex vivo. J Cell Biochem. 2012;113:658–668

19 Guilherme V. Silva, Silvio Litovsky, Joao A.R. Assad ed al. Mesenchymal Stem Cells Differentiate into an Endothelial Phenotype, Enhance Vascular Density, and Improve Heart Function in a Canine Chronic Ischemia Model. Circulation. 2005;111:150-156

20 Ning Yuan1, Wei Tian1, Lei Sun, et al., Neural stem cell transplantation in a double-layer collagen membrane with unequal pore sizes for spinal cord injury repair. Neural Regeneration Research. 2014; 9:10,1014-1019

21 Andrea Gärtner, Tiago Pereira, Raquel Gomes et al., Mesenchymal Stem Cells from Extra-Embryonic Tissues for Tissue Engineering – Regeneration of the Peripheral Nerve. "Advances in Biomaterials Science and Biomedical Applications" Chapter 18, March 27, 2013

22 Seaberg, R. M.; Van Der Kooy, D. "Stem and progenitor cells: The premature desertion of rigorous definitions." Trends in Neurosciences. 2003;26(3):125–131

23 Mason, John O.; Price, David J. "Building brains in a dish: Prospects for growing cerebral organoids from stem cells." Neuroscience. 2016; 334: 105–118

24 Bhartiya, D. Pluripotent Stem Cells in Adult Tissues: Struggling To Be Acknowledged Over Two Decades. Stem Cell Rev and Rep (2017) pp 1-12

25 Marks, P. W., Witten, C. M., & Califf, R. M. Clarifying stem cell therapy's benefits and risks. The New England Journal of Medicine, 2017; 376(11), 1007–1009

26 Singer NG, Caplan AI. Mesenchymal stem cells: mechanisms of inflammation. Annu Rev Pathol. 2011;6:457–78

27 Caplan AI. Mesenchymal stem cells. J Orthop Res. 1991;9:641–50

28 Volarevic V. et al., Bio-Factors, 2018, in press

29 Gnecchi M, Melo LG. Bone marrow-derived mesenchymal stem cells: isolation, expansion, characterization, viral transduction, and production of conditioned medium. Methods Mol Biol. 2009;482:281–294

30 Zhang X, Hirai M, Cantero S, Ciubotariu R, et al. Isolation and characterization of mesenchymal stem cells from human umbilical cord blood: reevaluation of critical factors for successful isolation and high ability to proliferate and differentiate to chondrocytes as compared to mesenchymal stem cells from bone marrow and adipose tissue. J Cell Biochem. 2011;112:1206–1218

31 Gimble J, Katz A, Bunnel B. Adipose-Derived Stem Cells for Regenerative Medicine. Circulation Research. 2007;100:1249-1260

32 Da Silva Meirelles L, Chagastelles PC, Nardi NB. Mesenchymal stem cells reside in virtually all post-natal organs and tissues. J Cell Sci 2006; 119: 2204–2213

33 Anker, P.S., Scherjon, S.A., Kleijburg-van der Keur, C., et al. (2003) Amniotic fluid as a novel source of mesenchymal stem cells for therapeutic transplantation. Blood 102, 1548–1549

34 Sessarego N, Parodi A, Podesta` M, Benvenuto F, Mogni M, Raviolo V et al. Multipotent mesenchymal stromal cells from amniotic fluid: solid perspectives for clinical application. Haematologica 2008; 93:339–346

35 Batsali AK, Kastrinaki MC, Papadaki HA, Pontikoglou C. Mesenchymal stem cells derived from Wharton's Jelly of the umbilical cord: biological properties and emerging clinical applications. Current stem cell research & therapy. 2013; 8: 144-155

36 Ishige I, Nagamura-Inoue T, Honda MJ, Harnprasopwat R, Kido M, Sugimoto M, Nakauchi H, Tojo A. Comparison of mesenchymal stem cells derived from arterial, venous, and Wharton's jelly explants of human umbilical cord. Int J Hematol. 2009;90:261–269

37 X.-J. Liang, X.-J. Chen, D.-H. Yang, S.-M. Huang, G.-D. Sun, and Y.-P. Chen, "Differentiation of human umbilical cord mesenchymal stem cells into hepatocyte-like cells by hTERT gene transfection in vitro," Cell Biology International, vol. 36, no. 2, pp. 215–221, 2012

38	Kern S, Eichler H, Stoeve J, Klüter H, Bieback K. Comparative analysis of mesenchymal stem cells from bone marrow, umbilical cord blood, or adipose tissue. Stem cells. 2006; 24: 1294-1301
39	Arirachakaran A, Sukthuayat A, Sisayanarane T, et al. Platelet-rich plasma versus autologous blood versus steroid injection in lateral epicondylitis: a systematic review and network meta-analysis. J Orthop Traumatol. 2016 Jun; 17(2):101-12
40	Foster TE, Puskas BL, Mandelbaum BR, Gerhardt MB, Rodeo SA. "Platelet-rich plasma: from basic science to clinical applications." Am J Sports Med. 2009; 37 (11): 2259–72
41	Frautschi, RS; Hashem, AM; Halasa, B; Cakmakoglu, C; Zins, JE (1 March 2017). "Current Evidence for Clinical Efficacy of Platelet Rich Plasma in Aesthetic Surgery: A Systematic Review.". Aesthetic surgery journal. 37 (3): 353–362
42	Bennell KL, Paterson L, Metcalf BR, et al. Effect of Intra-articular Platelet-Rich Plasma vs. Placebo Injection on Pain and Medial Tibial Cartilage Volume in Patients with Knee Osteoarthritis. JAMA. 2021;326(20):2021-2030. doi:10.1001/jama.2021.19415
43	Catlin S, Busque L, Gaile R at al. (Aril 2011) The replication of human hematopoietic stem cells in vitro. Blood, 117(17):4460-66
44	Murphy MB1, Blashki D, Buchanan RM Adult and umbilical cord blood-derived platelet-rich plasma for mesenchymal stem cell proliferation, chemotaxis, and cryopreservation. Biomaterials. 2012 Jul;33(21):5308-16
45	Serakinci N, Graakjaer J, Kolvraa S. Telomere stability and telomerase in mesenchymal stem cells. Biochimie. 2008; 90: 33-40
46	Tollervey JR, Lunyak VV. Adult stem cells: simply a tool for regenerative medicine or an additional piece in the puzzle of human aging? Cell Cycle 2011; 10: 4173–4176
47	Pipes BL, Tsang T, Peng SX, et al. Telomere length changes after umbilical cord blood transplant. Transfusion. 2006 Jun;46(6):1038-43
48	Mueller SM, Glowacki J. Age-related decline in the osteogenic potential of human bone marrow cells cultured in three-dimensional collagen sponges. J Cell Biochem. 2001;82:583–590
49	Campisi J, Cancer, aging, and cellular senescence. In Vivo. 2000 Jan-Feb; 14(1):183-8
50	Juhyun Oh, Yang David Lee et al. Stem cell aging: mechanisms, regulators and therapeutic opportunities. Nat Med. 2014 Aug 6; 20(8): 870–880
51	Organicel Regenerative Medicine, Inc
52	Park EH, White GA, Tieber LM. Mechanisms of injury and emergency care of acute spinal cord injury in dogs and cats. J Vet Emerg Crit Care (San Antonio). 2012;22(2):160-178
53	Godwin EE, Young NJ, Dudhia J, Beamish IC, Smith RK. Implantation of bone marrow-derived mesenchymal stem cells demonstrates improved outcome in horses with overstrain injury of the superficial digital flexor tendon. Equine Vet J. 2012;44(1):25-32
54	Cuervo B, Rubio M, Sopena J, et al. Hip osteoarthritis in dogs: a randomized study using mesenchymal stem cells from adipose tissue and plasma rich in growth factors. Int J Mol Sci. 2014;15(8):13437-13460
55	Harman R, Carlson K, Gaynor J, et al. A prospective, randomized, masked, and placebo-controlled efficacy study of intraarticular allogeneic adipose stem cells for the treatment of osteoarthritis in dogs. Front Vet Sci. 2016 Sep 16;3:81
56	Beerts C, Suls M, Broeckx SY, et al. Tenogenically induced allogeneic peripheral blood mesenchymal stem cells in allogeneic platelet-rich plasma: 2-year follow-up after tendon or ligament treatment in horses. Front Vet Sci. 2017;4:158

57	Van Loon VJ, Scheffer CJ, Genn HJ, Hoogendoom AC, Greve JW. Clinical follow-up of horses treated with allogeneic equine mesenchymal stem cells derived from umbilical cord blood for different tendon and ligament disorders. Vet Q. 2014;34(2):92-97
58	Herberts CA1, Kwa MS, Hermsen HP Risk factors in the development of stem cell therapy. J.Transl. Med. 2011;9:29
59	Marks, P. W., Witten, C. M., & Califf, R. M. Clarifying stem cell therapy's benefits and risks. The New England Journal of Medicine, 2017; 376(11), 1007–1009
60	"The Nobel Prize in Physiology or Medicine – 2012 Press Release". Nobel Media AB. 8 October 2012
61	Hockemeyer D, Jaenisch R (May 2016). "Induced Pluripotent Stem Cells Meet Genome Editing." Cell Stem Cell. 18 (5): 573–86
62	Knoepfler, Paul S. (2009). "Deconstructing Stem Cell Tumorigenicity: A Roadmap to Safe Regenerative Medicine." Stem Cells. 27 (5): 1050–1056
63	Arbuck DM, Current Psych. December 2021, 35-41 doi:10.12788/cp0192
64	Berkowitz AL et al. New England Journal of Medicine 2016 Jul 14;375(2):196-8
65	Rosemann A (Dec 2014). "Why regenerative stem cell medicine progresses slower than expected." J Cell Biochem. 115 (12): 2073–76
66	https://www.ecfr.gov/cgi-bin/retrieveECFR?gp=&SID=ff69887f399bdceb2b1f8ddaef-4d579e&mc=true&n=pt21.8.1271&r=PART&ty=HTML#se21.8.1271_145
67	https://www.fda.gov/news-events/press-announcements/fda-puts-company-notice-marketing-unapproved-stem-cell-products-treating-serious-conditions
68	https://www.fda.gov/inspections-compliance-enforcement-and-criminal-investigations/warning-letters/predictive-biotech-608322-08172020
69	https://www.fda.gov/vaccines-blood-biologics/consumers-biologics/important-patient-and-consumer-information-about-regenerative-medicine-therapies
70	https://www.fda.gov/news-events/press-announcements/fda-acts-remove-unproven-potentially-harmful-treatment-used-stem-cell-centers-targeting-vulnerable
71	www.mesoblast.com
72	Thirumala, S., Goebel, W.S. and Woods, E.J. (2009) Clinical grade adult stem cell banking. Organogenesis 5, 143–154
73	Gruen L, Grabel L. Concise review: scientific and ethical roadblocks to human embryonic stem cell therapy. Stem Cells 2006;24(10):2162–2169
74	Saha P, Sharma S, Korutla L et al. Circulating exosomes derived from transplanted progenitor cells aid the functional recovery of ischemic myocardium. Science Translational Medicine 2019 May 22 ; 11 (493), eaau1168
75	Zambelli A, Poggi G, Da Prada G, et al.,(1998) Clinical toxicity of cryopreserved circulating progenitor cells infusion. Anticancer Res 18:4705–8
76	Bissoyi A, Pramanik K. Role of the apoptosis pathway in cryopreservation-induced cell death in mesenchymal stem cells derived from umbilical cord blood. Biopreserv Biobank 2014;12:246-254
77	Yuan C, Gao J, Guo J, et al. (2014) Dimethyl Sulfoxide Damages Mitochondrial, Integrity and Membrane Potential in Cultured Astrocytes. PLoS ONE 9(9): e107447
78	Quintanar N., Patel R., Jones C., Importance of development of non-DMSO containing preservatives Progenokine Process and the effects of Cellular Viability from Umbilical Cord Blood Adherent Cells. Department of Research and Development, Burst Biologics, 2017

79 Holm F, Stro S, Inzunz J. (March 2010), An effective serum- and xeno-free chemically defined freezing procedure for human embryonic and induced pluripotent stem cells Reproduct Biol. 25 (5): 1271–79, 201

80 Weng JY, Du X, Geng SX, Peng YW, et al. Mesenchymal stem cell as salvage treatment for refractory chronic GVHD. Bone Marrow Transplant. 2010;45:1732–1740

81 Le Blanc K, Frassoni F, Ball L, et al. Mesenchymal stem cells for treatment of steroid-resistant, severe, acute graft-versus-host disease: a Phase II study. Lancet 2008;371(9624):1579–1586

82 Ringden O, Uzunel M, Rasmusson I, et al. Mesenchymal stem cells for treatment of therapy-resistant graft-versus-host disease. Transplantation 2006;81(10):1390–1397

83 Gonzales-Portillo GS, Sanberg PR, et al. Mannitol-Enhanced Delivery of Stem Cells and Their Growth Factors Across the Blood-Brain Barrier. Cell Transplant. 2014; 23(0): 531–539

84 Tajiri N, Lee JY, Acosta S, Sanberg PR, Borlongan CV. Breaking the Blood-Brain Barrier With Mannitol to Aid Stem Cell Therapeutics in the Chronic Stroke Brain. Cell Transplant. 2016; 25(8):1453-60

85 Brightman MW, Hori M, Rapoport SI, et al. Osmotic opening of tight junctions in cerebral endothelium. J Comp Neurol. 1973;152(4):317–325

86 Timbie KF, Mead BP, Price RJ: Drug and gene delivery across the blood-brain barrier with focused ultrasound. J Control Release. 2015;219:61–75

87 Meairs S: Facilitation of Drug Transport across the Blood-Brain Barrier with Ultrasound and Microbubbles. Pharmaceutics. 2015;7(3):275–293

88 Rodriguez A, Tatter SB, Debinski W: Neurosurgical Techniques for Disruption of the Blood-Brain Barrier for Glioblastoma Treatment. Pharmaceutics. 2015;7(3):175–187

89 Gherardini L, Bardi G, Gennaro M, et al. Novel siRNA delivery strategy: a new "strand" in CNS translational medicine? Cell Mol Life Sci. 2014;71(1):1–20. 10

90 Yarnitsky D, Gross Y, Lorian A, et al. Increased BBB permeability by parasympathetic sphenopalatine ganglion stimulation in dogs. Brain Res. 2004;1018(2):236–240

91 Dereymaeker A, Gonsette R: An experimental permeabilization of the blood-brain barrier by electric field application. Eur Neurol. 1977;15(6):333–339

92 https://www.scientificamerican.com/article/3-human-chimeras-that-already-exist/

93 Imanishi D, Miyazaki Y, et al. Donor-derived DNA in Fingernails Among Recipients of Allogeneic Hematopoietic Stem Cell Transplants. Blood. 2007 Oct 1;110(7):2231-4

94 See Bernaudin F et al., Long-term results of related myeloablative stem cell transplantation to cure sickle cell disease. Blood. 2007;110:2749-2756. "Hematopoietic stem cell transplantation (HSCT) is the only curative therapy for sickle cell disease."

95 Feng J, Mantesso A, De Bari C, Nishiyama A, Sharpe PT. Dual origin of mesenchymal stem cells contributing to organ growth and repair. Proc Natl Acad Sci U S A. 2011;108:6503–8

96 Fufaeva E, Semenova J, Semenova N, Sidorin S. Dynamics of high mental function recovery in children after severe traumatic brain injury having umbilical cord blood cells therapy. Brain Inj. 2012;26:688-689

97 DMEnnis J, Götherström C, Le Blanc K, Davies JE. In vitro immunologic properties of human umbilical cord perivascular cells. Cytotherapy. 2008;10:174–181

98 Weiss ML, Anderson C, Medicetty S, et al. Immune properties of human umbilical cord Wharton's jelly-derived cells. Stem Cells. 2008;26:2865–2874

99 Figueroa, F.F., Carri´on, F., Villanueva, S. and Khoury, M. (2012) Mesenchymal Stem Cell treatment for autoimmune diseases: a critical review. Biol. Res. 45, 269–77

100. Furlani D, Ugurlucan M, Ong L, Bieback K, Pittermann E, Westien I, et al. Is the intravascular administration of mesenchymal stem cells safe? Mesenchymal stem cells and intravital microscopy. Microvascular Research. 2009; 77: 370-376
101. Krasnodembskaya A, Samarani G, Song Y, Zhuo H, Su X, et al. (2012) Human mesenchymal stem cells reduce mortality and bacteremia in gram-negative sepsis in mice in part by enhancing the phagocytic activity of blood monocytes. Am J Physiol Lung Cell Mol Physiol 302: L1003–1013
102. Krasnodembskaya A, Song Y, Fang X, Gupta N, Serikov V, et al. (2010) Antibacterial effect of human mesenchymal stem cells is mediated in part from secretion of the antimicrobial peptide LL-37. Stem Cells 28: 2229–2238
103. Xiaojia Huang, Kai Sun1, Yidan D. Zhao, et al., Human CD34+ Progenitor Cells Freshly Isolated from Umbilical Cord Blood Attenuate Inflammatory Lung Injury following LPS Challenge PLOS ONE February 2014;9(2)
104. Pierro M, Ionescu L, Montemurro T, Vadivel A, Weissmann G, et al. (2013) Short-term, long-term and paracrine effect of human umbilical cord-derived stem cells in lung injury prevention and repair in experimental bronchopulmonary dysplasia. Thorax 68: 475–484
105. Mao Q, Chu S, Ghanta S, Padbury JF, De Paepe ME (2013) Ex vivo expanded human cord blood-derived hematopoietic progenitor cells induce lung growth and alveolarization in injured newborn lungs. Respir Res 14: 37
106. Nakajima H, Uchida K, Guerrero AR, Watanabe S, Sugita D, Takeura N et al. Transplantation of mesenchymal stem cells promotes an alternative pathway of macrophage activation and functional recovery after spinal cord injury. J Neurotrauma 2012; 29: 1614–1625
107. Park JH, Kim DY, Sung IY, Choi GH, Jeon MH, Kim KK et al. Long-term results of spinal cord injury therapy using mesenchymal stem cells derived from bone marrow in humans. Neurosurgery 2012; 70: 1238–1247
108. Chevalier X. Intraarticular treatments for osteoarthritis: new perspectives. Curr Drug Targets. 2010 May;11(5):546-60. Review
109. John A. Anderson, Dianne Little, Alison P. Toth, et al. Stem Cell Therapies for Knee Cartilage Repair The American Journal of Sports Medicine PreView, November 12, 2013
110. Shin Y-S, JungRo Yoon J-R, KimIntra H-S, et al. Articular Injection of Bone MarrowDerived Mesenchymal Stem Cells Leading to Better Clinical Outcomes without Difference in MRI Outcomes from Baseline in Patients with Knee Osteoarthritis Knee Surg Relat Res 2018;30(3):206-214
111. Gruber HE. Hanley ENJ. Recent advances in disc cell biology. Spine 2003; 28: 186–193
112. Ganey T, Hutton WC, Moseley T, Hedrick M, Meisel H-J. Intervertebral disc repair using adipose tissue-derived stem and regenerative cells: experiments in a canine model. Spine 2009; 34: 2297–2304
113. Erwin WM, Islam D, Eftekarpour E, at al. Intervertebral Disc-Derived Stem Cells Implications for Regenerative Medicine and Neural Repair. SPINE 2013;38(3):211–216
114. www.DiscGenics.com
115. Schneider BJ, Hunt C, Conger A, et al. The effectiveness of intradiscal biologic treatments for discogenic low back pain: a systematic review. Spine J. 2021; S1529-9430(21)00831-7
116. Matta A, Zia Karim M, Gerami H., et al. A comparative study of mesenchymal stem cell transplantation and NTG-101 molecular therapy to treat degenerative disc disease. Scientific Reports (2021) 11:14804
117. Matta A and Erwin ME, Current status of the instructional clues provided by notochordal cells in novel disk repair strategy. Int J of Mol Sci, 2022, 23, 427

118 Zebardast N, Lickorish D, Davies JE. Human umbilical cord perivascular cells (HUCPVC): A mesenchymal cell source for dermal wound healing. Organogenesis. 2010;6:197–203

119 Conconi MT, Burra P, Di Liddo R, Calore C, Turetta M, Bellini S, Bo P, Nussdorfer GG, Parnigotto PP. CD105(+) cells from Wharton's jelly show in vitro and in vivo myogenic differentiative potential. Int J Mol Med. 2006;18:1089–1096

120 Chaudhuri B, Pramanik K. Key aspects of the mesenchymal stem cells (MSCs) in tissue engineering for in vitro skeletal muscle regeneration. Biotechnol Mol Biol Rev 2012; 7: 5–15

121 Chen L, Tredget EE, Wu PYG, Wu Y. Paracrine factors of mesenchymal stem cells recruit macrophages and endothelial lineage cells and enhance wound healing. PLoS One 2008; 3: e1886

122 Parekkadan B, Milwid JM. Mesenchymal stem cells as therapeutics. Annu Rev Biomed Eng 2010; 12: 87–117

123 Uysal AC, et al. Differentiation of adipose-derived stem cells for tendon repair. Methods Mol. Biol. 2011;702:443-51

124 Doorn J, van de Peppel J, van Leeuwen JPTM, Groen N, van Blitterswijk CA, de Boer J. Pro-osteogenic trophic effects by PKA activation in human mesenchymal stromal cells. Biomaterials 2011; 32: 6089–6098

125 Parekkadan B, Milwid JM. Mesenchymal stem cells as therapeutics. Annu Rev Biomed Eng 2010; 12: 87–117

126 Mohanty ST, Bellantuono I. Intrafemoral injection of human mesenchymal stem cells. Methods Mol Biol. 2013;976:131–41

127 Kawamoto A, Tkebuchava T, Yamaguchi J, Nishimura H, Yoon YS, et al. Intramyocardial transplantation of autologous endothelial progenitor cells for therapeutic neovascularization of myocardial ischemia. Circulation 2003;107: 461–468

128 Assmus B, Schachinger V, Teupe C, Britten M, Lehmann R, et al. Transplantation of Progenitor Cells and Regeneration Enhancement in Acute Myocardial Infarction (TOPCARE-AMI). Circulation 2002; 106: 3009–3017

129 Cselenya´k A, Pankotai E, Horva´th EM, Kiss L, Lacza Z. Mesenchymal stem cells rescue cardiomyoblasts from cell death in an in vitro ischemia model via direct cell-to-cell connections. BMC Cell Biol 2010; 11: 29

130 Lipinski MJ, Luger D, Epstein SE. Mesenchymal Stem Cell Therapy for the Treatment of Heart Failure Caused by Ischemic or Non-ischemic Cardiomyopathy: Immunosuppression and Its Implications. Handb Exp Pharmacol. 2017;243:329-353

131 www.mesoblast.com

132 American Academy of Neurology 2021 Annual Meeting, Abstract 604. Presented April 5, 2022

133 Shyu WC, Lin SZ, Chiang MF, Su CY, Li H Intracerebral peripheral blood stem cell (CD34+) implantation induces neuroplasticity by enhancing beta1 integrin-mediated angiogenesis in chronic stroke rats. J Neurosci 2006;26: 3444–3453

134 Muir KW, Sinden J, Miljan E, Dunn L. Intracranial delivery of stem cells. Transl Stroke Res. 2011 Sep;2(3):266-71

135 Woodworth C, Jenkins G, Barron J at al. Intramedullary cervical spinal mass after stem cell transplantation using an olfactory mucosal cell autograft CMAJ July 08, 2019 191 (27) E761-E764

136 Wang Y, He X, et al. Peptide Programmed Hydrogels as Safe Sanctuary Microenvironments for Cell Transplantation. Advanced Functional Materials 29;(51) Dec 2019

137 https://www.nbcnews.com/health/health-news/fda-wins-case-against-florida-stem-cell-clinic-harmed-three-n1013641
138 Weiss JN, Levy S, Malkin A. Stem Cell Ophthalmology Treatment Study (SCOTS) for retinal and optic nerve diseases: a preliminary report. Neural Regen Res 2015; 10:982-8
139 Weiss JN, Levy S, Benes SC. Stem Cell Ophthalmology Treatment Study (SCOTS) for retinal and optic nerve diseases: a case report of improvement in relapsing autoimmune optic neuropathy. Neural Regen Res 2015; 10:1507-15
140 Labrador-Velandia S, Alonso-Alonso ML, Alvarez-Sanchez S, et al. , Mesenchymal stem cell therapy in retinal and optic nerve diseases: An update of clinical trials. World J Stem Cells. 2016 Nov 26;8(11):376-383
141 Zhang C., Yang SJ, Wen Q. et al. Human-derived normal mesenchymal stem/stromal cells in anticancer therapies Journal of Cancer 2017; 8(1): 85-96
142 Zhao W, Ren G, Zhang L, et al. Efficacy of mesenchymal stem cells derived from human adipose tissue in inhibition of hepatocellular carcinoma cells in vitro. Cancer Biother Radiopharm. 2012; 27: 606-13
143 Matsuzuka T, Rachakatla RS, Doi C, et al. Human umbilical cord matrix-derived stem cells expressing interferon-β gene significantly attenuate bronchioloalveolar carcinoma xenografts in SCID mice. Lung Cancer. 2010; 70: 28-36
144 Goldstein RH, Reagan MR, Anderson K, et al. Human bone marrow-derived MSCs can home to orthotopic breast cancer tumors and promote bone metastasis. Cancer Res. 2010; 70
145 Chu Y, Tang H, Guo Y, et al. Adipose-derived mesenchymal stem cells promote cell proliferation and invasion of epithelial ovarian cancer. Exp Cell Res. 2015; 337: 16-27
146 Lalu MM, McIntyre L, Pugliese C, et al. Safety of cell therapy with mesenchymal stromal cells (SafeCell): a systematic review and meta-analysis of clinical trials. PLoS One. 2012; 7: e47559
147 Dong L, Pu Y, Zhang L, et al. Human umbilical cord mesenchymal stem cell-derived extracellular vesicles promote lung adenocarcinoma growth by transferring miR-410 Cell Death and Disease (2018) 9:218
148 Wu S, Ju GQ, Du T. et al. Microvesicles derived from human umbilical cord Wharton's jelly mesenchymal stem cells attenuate bladder tumor cell growth in vitro and in vivo. PLoS ONE 8, e61366 (2013)
149 Vickers R, Karsten E, Flood J, Lilischkis R, A preliminary report on stem cell therapy for neuropathic pain in humans Journal of Pain Research 2014;7: 255–263
150 Vallejo R, Tilley DM, Vogel L, Benyamin R. The role of glia and the immune system in the development and maintenance of neuropathic pain. Pain Pract. 2010;10(3):167–184
151 Guo W, Wang H, Zou S, et al. Bone marrow stromal cells produce long-term pain relief in rat models of persistent pain. Stem Cells. 2011;29(8):1294–1303
152 Sacerdote P, Niada S, Franchi S, et al. Systemic administration of human adipose-derived stem cells reverts nociceptive hypersensitivity in an experimental model of neuropathy. Stem Cells Dev. 2013;22(8):1252–1263
153 Franchi S, Valsecchi AE, Borsani E, et al. Intravenous neural stem cells abolish nociceptive hypersensitivity and trigger nerve regeneration in experimental neuropathy. Pain. 2012;153(4):850–861
154 https://www.intechopen.com/books/regenerative-medicine-and-tissue-engineering/dental-related-stem-cells-and-their-potential-in-regenerative-medicine
155 Nokhbatolfoghahaei H, Rad MR, Khani MM, et al., Application of bioreactors to improve functionality of bone tissue engineering constructs: A systematic review. Curr Stem Cell Res Ther. 2017 Aug 21

156 Mangione F, EzEldeen M, Bardet C, et al. Implanted Dental Pulp Cells Fail to Induce Regeneration in Partial Pulpotomies. J Dent Res. 2017 Aug 1

157 Bajestan MN, Rajan A, Edwards SP, et al. Stem cell therapy for reconstruction of alveolar cleft and trauma defects in adults: A randomized controlled, clinical trial. Clin Implant Dent Relat Res. 2017 Jun 28

158 Tobita M, et al. Periodontal tissue regeneration with adipose-derived stem cells. Tissue Eng. Part A. 2008;14(6):945-953

159 Wu DC, Goldman MP. A Prospective, Randomized, Double-blind, Split-face Clinical Trial Comparing the Efficacy of Two Topical Human Growth Factors for the Rejuvenation of the Aging Face. J Clin Aesthet Dermatol. 2017 May;10(5):31-35

160 Ji J, Ho BS, Qian G, Xie XM, Bigliardi PL, Bigliardi-Qi MAging in hair follicle stem cells and niche microenvironment. J Dermatol. 2017 Jun 8

161 Deng W, et al. Mesenchymal stem cells regenerate skin tissue. Tissue Engineering. 2005;11:110-9

162 Mansilla, E et al., A Rat Treated with Mesenchymal Stem Cells Lives to 44 Months of Age. Rejuvenation Res. 2016 Aug 1; 19(4): 318–321

163 Zhang, B., Ma, S., Rachmin, I. et al. Hyperactivation of sympathetic nerves drives depletion of melanocyte stem cells. Nature 577, 676–681 (2020)

164 Segel M, Neumann BM, Hill M, et al. Niche stiffness underlies the ageing of central nervous system progenitor cells Nature (August 14, 2019)

165 Goodell, M. A. & Rando, T. A. Stem cells and healthy aging. Science (2015)350, 1199–1204

166 Geissler S, Textor M, Kuhnisch J, Konnig D, Klein O, et al. (2012) Functional comparison of chronological and in vitro aging: differential role of the cytoskeleton and mitochondria in mesenchymal stromal cells. PLoS One 7: e52700

167 Izadpanah R, Kaushal D, Kriedt C, Tsien F, Patel B, et al. (2008) Long-term in vitro expansion alters the biology of adult mesenchymal stem cells. Cancer Res 68: 4229–4238

168 Akita S, Hayashida K, Takaki S, et al. The neck burn scar contracture: a concept of effective treatment. Burns Trauma. 2017 Jul 13;5:22

169 Zhao B, Zhang Y, Han S, Zhang W et al., Exosomes derived from human amniotic epithelial cells accelerate wound healing and inhibit scar formation. J Mol Histol. 2017 Apr;48(2):121-132

170 Spiekman M, van Dongen JA, Willemsen JC et al. The power of fat and its adipose-derived stromal cells: emerging concepts for fibrotic scar treatment. J Tissue Eng Regen Med. 2017 Feb 3

171 Sorg H, Tilkorn DJ, Hager S, Hauser J, Skin Wound Healing: An Update on the Current Knowledge and Concepts. Eur Surg Res. 2017;58(1-2):81-94

172 Papanna et al. Cryopreserved Human Umbilical Cord Patch for In-utero Myeloschisis Repair. Obstet Gynecol, 128:325-30, 2016

173 Courtesy Scheffer Tseng, MD

174 Fufaeva E, Semenova J, Semenova N, Sidorin S. Dynamics of high mental function recovery in children after severe traumatic brain injury having umbilical cord blood cells therapy. Brain Inj. 2012;26:688-689

175 Dawson G, Sun L.M., Davlantis K., et al., Autologous Cord Blood Infusions Are Safe and Feasible in Young Children with Autism Spectrum Disorder: Results of a Single-Center Phase I Open-Label Trial. Stem Cells Translational Medicine. 2017;6:1332–1339

176 Shahaduzzaman M, Golden JE, Green S, et al. A single administration of human umbilical cord blood T cells produces longlasting effects in the aging hippocampus. Age (Dordr) 2013;35:2071–2087

177 Cotten CM, Murtha AP, Goldberg RN et al. Promising Therapies for Alzheimer's Disease

178 Confaloni A, Tosto G, Tata AM. Curr Pharm Des. 2016;22(14):2050-6 Feasibility of autologous cord blood cells for infants with hypoxic-ischemic encephalopathy. J Pediatr 2014;164:973–979.e1

179 Yedy I, Ezquer F, Quintanilla ME at al. Intracerebral Stem Cell Administration Inhibits Relapse-like Alcohol Drinking in Rats. Alcohol and Alcoholism, January 2017;52(1): 1–4

180 https://clinicaltrials.gov/ct2/show/NCT01534624

181 Arbuck DM, Current Psych. December 2021, 35-41 doi:10.12788/cp0192, already used as a reference in the iPSC section

182 https://www.cancer.gov/publications/dictionaries/cancer-terms/def/cytokine-storm

183 https://www.nytimes.com/interactive/2020/science/coronavirus-drugs-treatments.html

184 Ye Q, Wang B, et al. The pathogenesis and treatment of the Cytokine Storm in COVID-19. Journ of Infect. April, 2020, 80;(6): 607-613

185 https://celltrials.org/news/role-msc-treat-coronavirus-pneumonia-and-ards-part-1-is-emperor-wearing-clothes

186 https://clinicaltrials.gov/ct2/results?term=stem+cell&cond=COVID-19&age_v=&gndr=&type=&rslt=&phase=0&phase=1&phase=2&phase=3&Search=Apply

187 Ali Golchin A, Seyedjafari E, et al. Mesenchymal Stem Cell Therapy for COVID-19: Present or Future. Stem Cell Rev Rep. 2020 Jun;16(3):427-433

188 www.clinicaltrials.gov (NCT04486001)

189 Franctz C, Stewart KM, et al. The extracellular matrix at a glance. J Cell Sci 2010 Dec 15;123(24),4195-4200

190 Lim JJ, Koob TJ, Placental Cells and Tissues: The transformative rise in advanced wound care. Worldwide Wound Healing – innovation in natural and conventional methods (da Fonseca CJV, ed), 2016

191 Harrison, S. et al. Platelet activation by collagen provides sustained release of anabolic cytokines. Am J Sports Med 39, 729-734, doi:10.1177/0363546511401576 (2011)

192 Roberts DE, McNicol A, at al. Mechanism of collagen activation in human platelets. J Biol Chem 279, 19421-19430, doi:10.1074/jbc.M308864200 (2004)

193 Toyoda, T. et al. Direct activation of platelets by addition of CaCl2 leads coagulation of platelet-rich plasma. Int J Implant Dent 4, 23, doi:10.1186/s40729-018-0134-6 (2018)

194 Cavallo, C. et al. Platelet-Rich Plasma: The Choice of Activation Method Affects the Release of Bioactive Molecules. Biomed Res Int 2016, 6591717, doi: 10.1155/2016/6591717 (2016)

195 Iio, K. et al. Hyaluronic acid induces the release of growth factors from platelet-rich plasma. Asia Pac J Sports Med Arthrosc Rehabil Technol 4, 27-32, doi: 10.1016/j.asmart.2016.01.001 (2016)

196 Tada S, Kitajima T, et al. Design and synthesis of binding growth factors. Int J Mol Sci 13, 6053-6072, doi: 10.3390/ijms13056053 (2012)

197 Tollemar, V. et al. Stem cells, growth factors and scaffolds in craniofacial regenerative medicine. Genes Dis 3, 56-71, doi: 10.1016/j.gendis.2015.09.004 (2016)

198 De Witte TM, Fratila-Apachitei LE, at al. Bone tissue engineering via growth factor delivery: from scaffolds to complex matrices. Regen Biomater 5, 197-211, doi:10.1093/rb/rby013 (2018)

175	Gratwohl A et al., One million hematopoietic stem cell transplants: a retrospective observational study, Lancet Haematology 2, e91-e100, March 2015
200	Ballen KK, Gluckman E, Broxmeyer HE, Umbilical cord blood transplantation: the first 25 years and beyond, Blood. 122:491-498, 2013
201	Press release: "The Lancet Hematology: Experts warn of stem cell underuse as transplants reach 1 million worldwide" (Feb 26, 2016) http://www.eurekalert.org/pub_releases/2015-02/tl-tlh022515.php
202	Zhang J, Huang X, Wang H, Liu X, Zhang T, Wang Y, Hu D. The challenges and promises of allogeneic mesenchymal stem cells for use as a cell-based therapy. Stem Cell Res Ther. 2015 Dec 1;6:234. Review
203	Baraniak P., McDevitt T., Stem cell paracrine action and tissue regeneration Regen Med 2010 Jan; 5(1):121-143

Index

A

abdominal, 25, 73
aberrant differentiation, 15, 34, 69
accountability, 37
acellular, 3, 5, 26, 63-64, 68-70, 77-81, 90-91
Achilles tendon, 64
acupuncture, 55, 91
addiction, 74
adipose tissue, 18, 90-91
adult stem cell, 13, 15-16, 18, 21, 25, 38, 46-47, 55, 69, 81, 90-91
adverse effects, 28, 47, 53-54
aging, 1, 15, 24-25, 55, 71-72
alcohol, 74
allogeneic, 15-16, 21, 31, 35, 42, 47, 56, 62-63, 65, 76, 81, 84-85, 88-91
allograft, 70, 78-80, 84, 92-93
ALS, 59
Alzheimer's, 49, 59, 74
amniotic fluid, 3, 15, 20, 23, 42, 69, 77-79, 81, 84
amniotic membrane, 19-20, 78-79, 81, 84, 92-93
amplification, 27
animal, 1, 31, 35-37, 41, 44, 72-73, 84-85, 93
animal research, 31
animal stem cell, 31, 41, 84
anti-inflammatory process, 18, 84
Arnold Caplan, 16, 85
arthritis, 1, 9, 21, 38, 53, 56
asthma, 9, 27
asymmetric division, 11
atherosclerosis, 9
autism, 8-9, 74, 85
autoimmune, 1, 3-4, 8, 10, 16, 30, 56, 61, 85, 90-91
autologous, 15-17, 19, 21, 23, 31, 42, 46-47, 63, 66, 81, 84, 88-91

B

bacterial, 44
banking, 42, 85
biomaterial, 38
birth material, 14, 34, 36, 44
birth waste, 3, 5, 20, 24-25, 36, 38-39, 43, 45, 77, 79-80, 84, 90-91
blastocyst, 13, 84
blood bank, 39, 43-44, 85, 93
blood vessels, 9, 12, 47
bone, 8-9, 12-13, 15-18, 31, 38, 44, 46, 49, 55, 58, 60, 64, 80, 84-88, 90-91
bone fracture, 64
bone marrow, 8, 15-18, 31, 38, 44, 46, 49, 80, 84-85, 87, 90-91
bovine serum, 44
brain, 3-4, 12, 47-49, 59, 65-67, 72, 74, 85
bulging disc, 58

C

c-section, 5, 31, 36
cancer, 2, 9, 12, 15, 21, 28, 35-37, 42, 48, 56, 66, 69, 84-85, 87-88
cardiac, 65, 88
cartilage, 12-13, 23, 55-56, 59-60, 84
cat, 31
cell-to-cell interaction, 9, 90-91
cellular parts, 12
cellular survival, 46
cerebrospinal, 58-59
chemical influences, 45
chemoreceptors, 10
chromosome, 24-25, 49
chronic, 3-4, 37, 43, 53, 65, 80
collagen, 23, 79, 86
complications, 34-35, 71, 91
concentrate, 20, 23-25, 30, 34, 46, 59, 63, 69, 79
concerns, 8, 33-37, 66, 82, 84
connective tissue, 13, 17-18, 20-21, 23, 30, 52-53, 61-62, 77, 84
contamination, 36-37, 46
coronavirus, 40, 74-75
cosmetic, 71
cost, 37, 44, 90-91
counting stem cells, 45
COVID, 5, 40, 45, 54, 74-77, 80, 85
Crohn's disease, 9, 25, 56
cross-species, 31, 35, 41
crowding, 26, 45
cryopreservation, 14, 46
cupping, 55, 91
cure, 1, 4, 21, 25, 52-53, 55, 76, 85
cytokines, 4, 9-10, 20, 22-25, 27-29, 31, 34, 41, 44, 68, 74-76, 78-79, 84, 86, 88, 90-93
cytotoxic, 46

D

degenerative disc disease, 53, 58, 61-62
degenerative joint disease, 59
dementia, 48, 74
dental, 70
depression, 9, 74
destination, 10, 37, 59
diabetes, 8, 49, 65, 85
diet, 54
difference in opinion, 81
differentiation, 13, 15, 21, 34-35, 61, 69, 75-76, 87
dimethyl sulfoxide, 46
disc tear, 58, 61
discogenic cell, 62
disease transmission, 34
distribution, 29-30, 37, 42
divide, 11, 21, 24-26, 56
DMSO, 24-25, 46
DNA, 15, 26, 34, 44, 47-49

dog, 31
donating stem cells, 42
donor, 15, 19, 23, 36-37, 42, 44, 48-49, 53, 78, 84, 90-93
dose, 1-2, 4, 30, 47, 54-55, 58, 91
dry ice, 46
duration, 55

E

egg count, 56
embryo, 8, 13, 20, 34-35, 43, 84-85, 90-91
embryonic stem cell, 1, 20, 35-37, 41, 69, 84, 90-91
endocrine, 12-13, 55, 84
enhancement, 37
environment, 4, 12, 15, 27-28, 45, 55-56, 60-61, 66-67, 82, 84
epidural, 58, 91
ESC, 35-36
ethical, 8, 35-38, 40, 42-43, 84
exosomes, 1, 3-5, 7, 9, 11, 13, 15, 17, 19-21, 23-25, 27-31, 33-35, 37, 39, 41-42, 45, 47, 49, 51, 53, 55, 57, 59, 61, 63, 65, 67-69, 71, 73, 75, 77-79, 81, 83-85, 87, 89-91, 93
expansion, 37, 41
expensive, 15, 21, 34, 37, 39-40, 44, 46
extracellular, 5, 10, 16, 22, 28, 57, 65, 71, 77-80, 84, 92-93

F

fat, 12-13, 15, 17, 31, 58, 71
FDA, 14, 20, 38-42, 46, 52-53, 62, 65, 68, 78, 80, 82, 85-86, 88-89, 92-93
federal funding, 38
federal guidelines, 42
flu-like sensation, 53, 91
freezing, 45-46, 68

G

glycerol, 46-47
God, 34-35
graft, 14, 16, 46-47
graft-versus-host disease, 47
growing organs, 73
growth factors, 4, 9-10, 20, 22, 24, 27-28, 34, 41, 44, 61, 63, 68, 70-71, 78-79, 84, 87, 90-93
gut, 3-4, 56

H

hair, 71-73
harvesting stem cell, 19, 31
heart, 3, 9-10, 12, 29, 41, 48, 53, 65, 87-88
hematopoiesis, 8, 85, 87
hematopoietic stem cell, 13, 15-16, 18, 39, 84, 93
herniated disc, 61
hidden danger, 3
history, 4, 8, 53, 85
HLA, 16-17, 44
homing, 10, 65
horse, 31
human, 1, 16, 21, 24-25, 29, 31, 34, 36, 40-41, 45, 47, 62, 68, 71, 76, 78, 80-81, 85-86, 88-89, 92-93

human embryonic stem cell, 1, 41
human leukocyte antigens, 16
hyaline cartilage, 23

I

immune compatibility, 16
immune conflict, 16
immune markers, 15-16
immune reaction, 34
immune regulation, 18, 76
immune system, 1, 10, 16, 18, 20, 23, 34, 47-48, 60-61, 69, 74, 84-85, 88
immunologic, 44
immunosuppression, 2, 16, 47-48
in vivo, 23
induction of stem cells, 23
infertility, 56
inflammation, 1, 9, 18, 23, 25, 38, 47, 54, 59, 62, 67-69, 74-76, 78-79, 84, 91
inflammatory bowel disease, 9
infusion, 10, 14, 22, 25, 43, 48, 52-54, 58, 65-66, 71, 76, 91
interstitial cystitis, 56
intra-articular, 23
intracardiac, 65
intradiscal, 61-62
intraligament, 64
intramuscular, 22, 63
intraocular, 48, 68
intraorgan, 65
intraosseous, 64
intraspinal, 65-66
intrathecal, 48, 58-59, 67, 91
intrauterine surgery, 19
intraventricular, 66

J

joint, 4, 10, 21-22, 24-25, 38, 52-54, 58-60, 91

K

kidney, 3, 46, 48, 53, 65, 85
knee, 3-4, 23, 38-39, 53, 59-60, 64

L

labrum, 59
lidocaine, 45, 54, 56
ligament, 13, 22, 46, 64, 79, 84
liquid biopsy, 45
liquid nitrogen, 46
longevity, 57, 72
low back, 3, 58, 62
lung, 3, 43, 48, 53, 56-57, 60, 76, 85
lupus, 56
lyme disease, 56
lymphocyte, 18, 76, 84
lysosome, 27

M

macrophage, 18, 74, 76, 84, 86
major histocompatibility complex, 16
manipulation, 1, 37, 41-42, 73, 88-89
marketing, 26, 28, 40
matrix, 5, 9, 22, 61, 63, 71, 77-81, 84, 87, 90-93
mature cell, 13, 36, 90-91
mental illness, 74
mesenchymal stem cell, 12, 14-18, 30, 45, 62, 75-76, 84-85, 93
MHC, 16
migration, 22, 49, 63, 65, 87-88
miracle, 4, 35, 38
mitochondria, 12, 25, 27
mitochondrial transfer, 9, 12
mixing stem cells, 42
monocyte, 18, 84
moral, 35-36, 84
moxibustion, 55, 91
Multiple Sclerosis, 53, 59, 66
multiply, 19, 22, 44, 56, 71
muscle, 10, 12-13, 22, 46, 52-54, 63, 84
musculoskeletal system, 31
mutation, 21, 26, 34, 44, 46-47
Myasthenia gravis, 56-57
Myer's cocktail, 53

N

nasal, 66, 68
neck, 3, 61
needle, 1, 45, 53, 71
neoplasia, 21
nerve cells, 12, 61
nerve tissue, 12
nervous system, 9, 47-48, 59, 66, 87
neurons, 12, 47, 87
nucleus pulposus, 61
number of treatments, 55

O

oncogenesis, 21, 36, 84
organ, 10-11, 18-19, 22, 27, 47-48, 53, 56, 65, 73, 84, 87-88
organ repair, 18, 84
osteoarthritis, 23, 38-39, 60, 80
outcomes, 3, 13, 23, 35-36, 52-53, 62-63, 65-66, 82
overdose, 28
overseas, 37, 42
oxygen, 9, 12, 43, 57, 61

P

packaging, 12
pain, 1, 3, 21, 23, 25, 35, 38, 52-54, 58-62, 69, 73, 91
pandemic, 45, 74, 76
Parkinson's, 59, 66

patient experience, 52-53, 91
pharmaceutical, 1, 40, 82
phenotype, 37
physical therapy, 54
placenta, 14, 20, 43, 63, 69-70, 77, 79-80, 90-91
plantar fasciitis, 64
plasma, 18, 22, 26, 80, 84
platelet-rich plasma, 22, 84
plexus, 12
post-menopausal, 23
post-treatment, 54
preconception, 34
precursor, 13, 15, 61, 65-66, 79, 84
preservation, 24-26, 34, 37, 42, 45-46, 78-79
processing, 30, 42, 44
progenitor stem cell, 13, 84
prolotherapy, 23
propagate, 22
prophylactic, 34, 57, 71, 76
proteins, 15, 22-23, 45, 66, 84, 86-87
PRP, 22-23, 46, 59, 63-64, 79-81, 84
psychosis, 9, 74
PT, 54, 91

R

radiation, 26, 47, 56, 78
rash, 1, 3, 61
regenerative biologics, 41, 91
regenerative medicine, 1, 3-5, 24-25, 28, 31, 39-41, 52-53, 63, 77, 80-82, 85
regenerative potential, 10, 14
regulation, 18, 34, 38-40, 43, 52-53, 62, 76, 78, 82, 85, 88-89
rejection, 16, 46-47
rejuvenate, 24-25, 71
relatives, 42
religious concern, 34-36, 84
repair, 1, 8-9, 12, 18-20, 22-25, 28, 30, 48, 52-53, 55, 58-59, 61, 64-65, 69, 73, 76, 79, 84, 87-88
repeated treatment, 37-38, 43, 55
replicate, 11
reprogramming, 36
resistant infection, 3
restriction, 37-38, 77
reward, 5, 34, 82
rheumatoid arthritis, 9, 56
ribosome, 27
risk, 2, 5, 10, 21, 29, 34, 37, 39, 42, 46-47, 66, 69, 82, 90-93
RNA, 15, 44

S

sacroiliac joint, 59
safety, 1, 16, 21, 24-25, 34, 36-42, 45-47, 52-53, 66, 69, 81-82
SARS, 74, 80
scaffolding, 18, 86
scar, 3, 19, 23, 53, 71, 73
sciatica, 58

screening, 37, 44
secreted factors, 10
senescence, 25
sensationalism, 36
shipment, 46
shoulder, 3-4, 21, 39, 61, 64
sickle cell anemia, 8, 85
skin, 1, 4, 36, 61-62, 71-73, 78-79
specialized cells, 11, 13
sperm, 56
spina bifida, 20, 73
spinal cord, 4, 58-59, 66
spinal discs, 12, 62
spinal root impingement, 58
spinal tumor, 66
spine facets, 59
spleen, 56
sports injury, 52-53, 64
stability, 46, 53, 80
stem cell matrix, 22
stem cell product, 14, 18, 20, 24-26, 31, 37, 39-40, 44, 64, 68-69, 81
stem cell research, 16, 31, 35, 38, 82
steroid, 1-2, 54, 56, 58
stimulant, 23, 28, 48, 74, 81
storage, 26, 30, 44, 46, 68, 78, 90-91
stress, 14, 47, 54, 72
survivability, 10, 34, 46, 59, 61, 67, 87
swelling, 12, 54, 91
symmetric division, 11
systemic reaction, 46

T

telomeres, 15, 24-25, 55
teratogenesis, 28
test, 16, 34, 37, 39, 42, 44-45, 53, 57, 82
thawing, 2, 14, 45-46, 53, 79
thymus, 10, 56
tissue bank, 39
tissue testing, 45
topical, 20, 71, 84
totipotent stem cell, 13, 84
toxin, 26, 47-48
tracking number, 53
transplantation, 8-10, 14-15, 21-22, 35, 45, 47-49, 54-56, 59, 61, 63, 65-67, 70, 76, 85
transverse myelitis, 59
traumatic brain injury, 59, 66, 74
travel abroad, 37-38
trophic factors, 10, 22
tumorigenesis, 15, 37, 66, 69, 90-91

U

umbilical cord blood stem cells, 3, 21, 27, 84, 93
umbilical cord stem cell, 1, 5, 13, 16, 18-19, 21, 24-25, 31, 36, 42, 47, 56, 61, 71, 76, 84, 93
umbilical cord wall, 3, 17, 21, 84

undifferentiated, 36, 84
unresolved inflammation, 9

V

vacuole, 28
vascularization, 12, 61
veterinary medicine, 31
viral, 44
vitality, 21, 26, 45-46, 56, 67, 71, 77, 90-91

W

waste, 3, 5, 20, 24-25, 27-28, 36, 38-39, 42-43, 45, 77, 79-80, 84, 90-91
Wharton's jelly, 14, 21, 69, 81, 85
wound, 3, 9, 19-20, 35, 73, 78, 84, 87-88

Made in the USA
Las Vegas, NV
22 August 2023

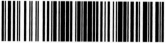